Home Health Care

Recent Titles in
Bibliographies and Indexes in Gerontology

Human Longevity from Antiquity to the Modern Lab: A Selected, Annotated Bibliography
William G. Bailey, compiler

Federal Public Policy on Aging since 1960: An Annotated Bibliography
William E. Oriol, compiler

European American Elderly: An Annotated Bibliography
David Guttmann, compiler

Legal Aspects of Health Care for the Elderly: An Annotated Bibliography
Marshall B. Kapp, compiler

Crime and the Elderly: An Annotated Bibliography
Ron H. Aday, compiler

Jewish Elderly in the English-Speaking Countries
David Guttmann, compiler

Women and Aging: A Selected, Annotated Bibliography
Jean M. Coyle, compiler

Fundamentals of Geriatrics for Health Professionals: An Annotated Bibliography
Jodi L. Teitelman and Iris A. Parham, compilers

Geriatric Nursing Assistants: An Annotated Bibliography with Models to Enhance Practice
George H. Weber

Anthropology of Aging: A Partially Annotated Bibliography
Marjorie M. Schweitzer, general editor

Families and Aging: A Selected, Annotated Bibliography
Jean M. Coyle, compiler

Pastoral Responses to Older Adults and Their Families: An Annotated Bibliography
Henry C. Simmons and Vivienne S. Pierce

HOME HEALTH CARE

An Annotated Bibliography

COMPILED BY

ADA ROMAINE-DAVIS
AYELIFFE A. LENIHAN
MOIRA D. SHANNON

Bibliographies and Indexes in Gerontology, Number 16
Erdman B. Palmore, Series Adviser

Greenwood Press
New York • Westport, Connecticut • London

Library of Congress Cataloging-in-Publication Data

Romaine-Davis, Ada.
Home health care : an annotated bibliography / compiled by Ada Romaine-Davis, Ayeliffe A. Lenihan, Moira D. Shannon.
p. cm.—(Bibliographies and indexes in gerontology, ISSN 0743-7560 ; no. 16)
Includes bibliographical references and indexes.
ISBN 0-313-28334-6 (alk. paper)
1. Home care services—Bibliography. I. Lenihan, Ayeliffe A. II. Shannon, Moira D. III. Title. IV. Series.
Z6675.H69R65 1992
[RA645.3]
016.3621'4—dc20 91-46848

British Library Cataloguing in Publication Data is available.

Library of Congress Catalog Card Number: 91-46848
ISBN: 0-313-28334-6
ISSN: 0743-7560

First published in 1992

Greenwood Press, 88 Post Road West, Westport, CT 06881
An imprint of Greenwood Publishing Group, Inc.

Printed in the United States of America

The paper used in this book complies with the Permanent Paper Standard issued by the National Information Standards Organization (Z39.48-1984).

10 9 8 7 6 5 4 3 2 1

Contents

Series Foreword

The annotated bibliographies in this series provide answers to the fundamental question, "What is known?" Their purpose is simple, yet profound: to provide comprehensive reviews and references for the work done in various fields of gerontology. They are based on the fact that it is no longer possible for anyone to comprehend the vast body of research and writing in even one sub-specialty without years of work.

This fact has become true only in recent years. When I was an undergraduate (Class of '52) I think no one at Duke had even heard of gerontology. Almost no one in the world was identified as a gerontologist. Now there are over 6,000 professional members of the Gerontological Society of America. When I was an undergraduate there were no courses in gerontology. Now there are thousands of courses offered by most major (and many minor) colleges and universities. When I was an undergraduate there was only one gerontological journal (the Journal of Gerontology, begun in 1945). Now there are over forty professional journals and several dozen books in gerontology published each year.

The reasons for this dramatic growth are well known: the dramatic increase in numbers of aged, the shift from family to public responsibility for the security and care of the elderly, the recognition of aging as a "social problem," and the growth of science in general. It is less well known that this explosive growth in knowledge has developed the need for new solutions to the old problem of comprehending and "keeping up" with a field of knowledge. The old indexes and library card catalogues have become increasingly inadequate for the job. On-line computer indexes and abstracts are one solution, but they make no evaluative selections nor organize sources logically as is done here. These annotated bibliographies are also more widely available than on-line computer indexes.

These bibliographies will obviously be useful for students and researchers who need to know what research has (or has not) been done in their field. The annotations contain enough information so that the researcher usually does not have to search out the original articles. In the past, the "review of literature" has often been haphazard and was rarely comprehensive, because of the large investment of time (and money) that would be required by a truly comprehensive review. Now, using these bibliographies, researchers can be more confident that they are not missing and "reinventing the wheel." It may well become standard and expected practice for researchers to consult such bibliographies, even before they start their research.

The area of home health care is one of the fastest growing in gerontology and geriatrics. One of the main reasons is economics. It is usually less expensive to provide home health care than institutionalization, unless the patient needs continuous nursing service. Thus, a major motivation for home health care is often cost control.

Another major reason for the growth in home health care is the general perference among patients to stay in their own home as long as possible. This usually has many advantages such as avoiding the trauma of moving and adapting to institutional life, being in familiar surroundings, being more in control of one's own regime and schedule, etc.

The rapid growth in home health care has been accompanied by rapid growth in research and writing about the field. Thus, a comprehensive bibliography in this area is one of the most useful and important tools in gerontology.

This book is needed not only by academics, researchers, and students, but also by health professionals and others who work with elders, as well as by elders themselves, their families, and anyone else interested in home health care.

The authors have done an outstanding job of covering all the recent literature and organizing it into easily accessible form. Not only are there 370 annotated references organized into 10 chapters and 10 sub-sections, there is also an introduction, a preface, an author index, and a subject index with many cross-references for the items in the bibliography.

Thus, one can look for relevant material in this volume in several ways: (1) look up a given subject in the subject index; (2) look up a given author in the author index; or (3) turn to the section that covers the topic.

The three authors of this bibliography are well qualified for the task. Not only are they registered nurses, but all three have earned doctorates in the field, and the senior author, Ada Romaine-Davis, is also a Certified Adult Nurse Practitioner.

So it is with great pleasure that we add this bibliography to our series. We believe you will find this volume to be the most useful, comprehensive, and easily accessible reference work in its field. I will appreciate any comments you care to send me.

Erdman B. Palmore
Center for the Study of Aging and Human Development
Box 3003, Duke University Medical Center
Durham, NC 27710

Preface

This book is intended to provide a relatively extensive, detailed, selected bibliography on the major aspects of home care for the elderly.

Included are 370 citations, primarily from the late 1980s to the present, thus making the contents as current as possible.

The references are to provide guideposts to additional relevant published material on this rapidly changing field. Annotations supply cogent information and results of research in sufficient detail for readers to grasp the scope and conclusions of the article or report.

Within each section, the items are alphabetized by name of first author. All citations are numbered consecutively from start to finish to facilitate access. All references are accessible from established library databases and government sources.

The chapter and section headings are perceived by the compilers as the most important issues in home care at this time. Health problems listed under "Care in the Home," for example, were chosen as being the most common seen in home care patients, those that pose the greatest challenge to caregivers, and those most amenable to preventive measures. Areas in which the literature revealed apparent paucities included prevention of chronic health problems and disability, legal issues, and selected ethical dilemmas such as rationing of available resources and over-medication. There were references to the ethical dilemmas of euthanasia, abuse, termination of life support, and suicide.

In the indexes, the numbers following each entry refer to the number of the citation, not the page number.

Acknowledgments

The compilers wish to acknowledge the assistance and support of, first, Dr. Erdman Palmore, series editor and, at Greenwood Press, Ms. Ann LeStrange, Assistant Managing Editor and, most especially, Dr. George F. Butler, Acquisitions Editor, Social and Behavioral Sciences, who provided specific and detailed directions regarding procedures and formatting of the manuscript. Andrew Schub, Assistant Production Editor, was most helpful in the final preparation of the book.

Second, librarians and staff members of libraries and organizations, including the Parklawn Library of the Public Health Service, Rockville, Maryland, McKeldin Graduate Library, the Health Sciences Library, and the Center for Aging at the University of Maryland, College Park and Baltimore, Education Resources Information Center (ERIC), and the National Home Care Association, Washington, DC.

Last, we want to publicly express our appreciation for the help and support provided by our husbands, John F. Davis, Robert E. Lenihan, and Kevin F. Arundel.

Introduction

Home health care (HHC) is emerging as a major component of the health care industry. As a dynamic force, home health care is currently experiencing both rapid growth and complex change.[1] Two primary factors are providing the impetus for both growth and change: economics, and the increasing number of older persons.

Costs of HHC services by all payers rose from $6 billion in 1985 to about $6.8 billion in 1988 and to $10.5 billion in 1990. Projected expenditures for 1995 are estimated to be $14.2 billion.[2] Because of the rapid increase in cost of health care in all settings, people are seeking care that is less costly and that also allows them to be as independent as possible and to retain control of decisions regarding their own care. For these reasons noninstitutional care, while not always significantly less expensive than institutional care, is preferred. Strides are being made, however, to make HHC more cost-effective. One way to do this is to employ case management methods to coordinate care and eliminate duplication of aspects of care. Ideally, one case manager coordinates continuous care as the client moves from home to hospital during an acute episode of illness, to nursing home for convalescence, and back to home for monitoring, prevention of complications, and promotion of health status.[3]

Along with increased utilization of HHC services, the growth of HHC agencies has been equally dramatic. The number of Medicare-certified HHC agencies increased from 1753 in 1967 to 5277 in 1987. In 1990, this number increased to 5721.[4] While individual agencies tend to be small, many are part of large, complex systems. Administrators therefore need to understand and apply managerial and financial principles in order to survive and prosper in the expanding competitive health care marketplace. Organizational structure, financial management, including reimbursement issues, and database development and maintenance, are part of the successful administrator's armamentarium. Important also is a firm knowledge base about Federal, state, and local legislation and regulations, quality assurance and accreditation issues and requirements, and sources of actual and potential support from both the public and private sectors. Governmental and organizational policies relating to HHC and HHC services continue to change rapidly.

Ethical and legal/malpractice issues and questions are evoking greater reaction and response from the perspectives of both clients and providers. Among these issues are euthanasia, withholding of treatment, pain management, over-medication, negligence, advance directives, and others. Both the administrator and the practitioner need up-to-date and accurate information about changes in these areas.

Many factors differentiate home and institutional care. Among these differences are the environment itself, available resources, differences in cultural and health perspectives in terms of how care is ordinarily given by family members, and the changed relationships and roles of clients and providers, with the provider being a guest in the home and thus lacking the level of perceived control that is usual when the client is in an institution or in the provider's office.

The role of the caregiver in providing care to the elderly has been studied from many perspectives. Caregivers are usually family members who provide ongoing, personal, unpaid service in a variety of ways. The burden that accompanies this role, the types of support needed and available, and the intergenerational issues that surface have all been described in the literature.

Evaluation of the agency, program, method of assignment of employees, treatment protocols, patient outcomes, and level of satisfaction are elements to be included in a comprehensive evaluation plan to ensure quality, efficiency, and cost-effectiveness of care.

Research data are sparse in many areas, including cost-benefits and effectiveness of HHC. Many researchers are currently concentrating their efforts on these types of studies. Much has been done in the last ten years, and much has been learned about the physiological and psychological aspects of aging, attitudes of elderly people and health care providers regarding the elderly, and levels and scope of care required in the home setting, based on individual and family needs. Integrated efforts and shared resources will help to coordinate and complement research activities, and to provide more rigorous studies that will produce more valid and reliable data in these vital areas.

This bibliography was compiled with these and other aspects of HHC in mind, to develop a comprehensive and valuable guide to the current literature for physicians, nurses, administrators, lawyers, policy planners, social workers, researchers, caregivers, families, clients, students and interested others.

References:

1. Woerner L., Feldstein K. C. (1988). Scheduling Home Health Care Personnel. New York: Wiley & Sons, vii.

2. National Association for Home Care (1987). Basic Statistics on Home Health Care, August. Washington, DC: NAHC.

3. Bernstein L. H., Grieco A. J., Dete M. K. (1987). Primary Care in the Home. Philadelphia: Lippincott, 66-67.

4. Prospective Payment Assessment Commission (1991). Medicare and the American Health Care System: Report to the Congress. Washington, DC: Prospective Payment Assessment Commission, June, 98.

Abbreviations

Adv Nurs Sci	Advances in Nursing Science
AIDS	Acquired Immuno-deficiency Syndrome
Amer J Publ Health	American Journal of Public Health
AoA	Administration on Aging
DNA	deoxyribonucleic acid; genetic molecules
EBRI	Employee Benefit Research Institute
ERIC	Educational Resources Information Center
Fam Community Health	Family and Community Health
Fam Relations	Family Relations

FDA	Food and Drug Administration
GAO	General Accounting Office
Geriatr Nurs	Geriatric Nursing
HCFA	Health Care Financing Administration
HIV	Human Immunodeficiency Virus
HIVAT	Home Intravenous Antibiotic Therapy
Holistic Nurs Pract	Holistic Nursing Practice
J Advanc Nurs	Journal of Advanced Nursing
J Aging & Health	Journal of Aging and Health
JAMA	Journal of the American Medical Association
J Amer Acad Nurs Pract	Journal of the American Academy of Nurse Practitioners
J Amer Geritr Soc	Journal of the American Geriatric Society
J Cancer Nurs	Journal of Cancer Nursing

J Fam Issues	Journal of Family Issues
J Geront Nurs	Journal of Gerontological Nursing
J Neurosci Nurs	Journal of Neuroscience Nursing
J Nurs Admin	Journal of Nursing Administration
J Nutr for Elderly	Journal of Nutrition for the Elderly
J Soc Serv Res	Journal of Social Service Research
LTC	Long Term Care
Med Care	Medical Care
NCA	National Council on Aging
NITA	National Institute for the Treatment of AIDS
NSAIDs	nonsteroidal anti-inflammatory drugs
NTIS	National Technical Information Service
Nurs Clin North Am	Nursing Clinics of North America
Nurs Res	Nursing Research
PIC	Policy Information Center

PPAC	Prospective Payment Assessment Commission
PPS	Prospective Payment System
Res Nurs & Health	Research in Nursing and Health
SHMO	Social Health Maintenance Organization
Soc Serv Rev	Social Service Review
Soc Work	Social Work
VNAAs	Visiting Nurses Associations of America

1

Overview

1. Ade-Ridder L., Hennon C. B. (eds.) (1989). Life-styles of the Elderly: Diversity in Relationships, Health, and Caregiving. New York: Human Sciences Press, Inc.

This book comprises three major sections: long-term marriages, family and friends, and importance of health. Many aspects of marriage are addressed: characteristics of couples married for 30 years or more, quality of marriage, family strengths in long-term marriages, factors affecting long-term marriage, retirement and marriage, and others. The middle section explores relationships of older couples with family and friends, grandparenthood, and teenagers' interaction with grandparents. The final section deals with maintenance of health over the later years, roles of spouse caregivers, and aspects of health problems within the context of the family. A comprehensive resource for those providing care of the elderly in the home.

2. Baines E.M. (ed.) (1991). Perspectives on Gerontological Nursing. Newbury Park, CA: Sage Publications.

This book is written by experts in the field of gerontological nursing and provides comprehensive information about both illness and wellness care of the elderly. Included in the book are chapters on physiological and psychological illnesses, rehabilitation of older persons, ethical and legal issues in aging, and cross-national trends in health care for the elderly.

3. Bergener M., Ermini M., Stahelin H. B. (eds.) (1989). Crossroads in Aging: The 1988 Sandoz Lectures in Gerontology. San Diego, CA: Academic Press.

There are two previous volumes to this one, and none is outdated. This issue stimulates scientific curiosity in aging beyond one's own discipline and promotes the search for additional knowledge in the challenging field of human aging.

4. Bergener M., Ermini M., Stahelin H. B. (eds.) (1991). Challenges in Aging: The 1990 Sandoz Lectures in Gerontology. San Diego, CA: Academic Press.

This book comprises the papers presented at the Sandoz Lectures conference. Three main areas are the focus: 1) Human Competence: Changes Under Normal and Pathological Conditions; 2) Regulatory Factors of Cell Function during Aging; and 3) Chronic Illness in the Elderly: Clinical Strategies. A summary of each topic area is provided, and general conclusions are summarized in the final section.

5. Bernstein C., Bernstein H. (1991). Aging, Sex, and DNA Repair. San Diego, CA: Academic Press.

The authors provide an integrated explanation of aging and sex, based on current knowledge about DNA damage and repair. Topics covered include: 1) Universality of the problem of DNA damage; 2) Aging as a consequence of accumulated DNA damage; 3) Meiosis as an adaptation for DNA repair; and 4) Mating, in eukaryotes, as an adaptation for masking mutation.

6. Binstock R. H., George L. K. (eds.) (1990). Handbook of Aging and the Social Sciences: Third Edition. San Diego, CA: Academic Press.

Updates on important issues examined in earlier editions are provided and cover new areas pertinent to the social aspects of aging. An international perspective is provided with several international authors contributing and many chapters presenting a review of international and cross-national research. New topics include: 1) Geographic distribution and migration; 2) Mortality and morbidity; 3) Leisure and time use across the life course; 4) Social structure, social processes, and social psychological states; 5) Illness behavior in later life; and 6) A comparative study of old-age pensions.

7. Birren J. E. et al (1991). The Concept and Measurement of Quality of Life in the Frail Elderly. San Diego, CA: Academic Press.

This is the first serious attempt to impose rigor on the definition and measurement of quality of life among the elderly. A conference is used to develop the background, but goes beyond that format in terms of literature reviews and coordination of topics. An excellent book for researchers in any discipline where there is inquiry being conducted in the area of well-being of the elderly.

8. Brannon D., Smyer M. A. (1990). Who will provide long-term care in the future? Generations:64-67, spring.

This article presents a thorough discussion of personnel projections to meet the growing long-term care needs of the future, both in nursing homes and in home health care agencies. The authors predict intensified competition for all levels and types of health care workers in all settings. Planning strategies to meet these needs are discussed. These projections have critical implications for the future of long-term care financing, administration of health care facilities and agencies, and quality of care.

9. Brickner P. W., Lechich A. J., Lipsman E., Scharer L. K. (1987). Long-Term Health Care. New York: Basic Books, Inc.

This reference work comprises major aspects regarding long-term care: growing need, financial problems, health problems, dementia, and a lengthy separate section on home care that highlights New York State's Long Term Home Health Care Program, quality of care, types of long-term care, and trends. Recommended for health professionals, health care financing experts, and policy planners.

10. Brody S. J., Pawlson G. L. (1990). Aging and Rehabilitation II: The State of the Practice. New York: Springer Publishing Company.

This book is the result of a national conference on aging and rehabilitation sponsored by the Bureau of Health Professions and the National Institute on Aging in December 1988. Eight aspects of aging and rehabilitation are highlighted: 1) basic issues in rehabilitation of the elderly, 2) autonomy of the disabled elderly, 3) the Practice Model (PM): Mobility, 4) PM: Environment, 5) PM: Continence, 6) PM: Mental Health, 7) PM: Assessment, and 8) Ethical and Values Issues. The need to develop a multidisciplinary geriatric rehabilitation team approach to education and practice is emphasized throughout.

11. Callahan D. (1990). What Kind of Life: The Limits of Medical Progress. New York: Simon and Schuster.

The individual versus the common good is explored in the context of costs of medical treatment, allocation of scarce resources, and the political and societal aspects of health care and expectations. Different approaches and strategies to change the current and future health care system are presented. This is a reality-oriented perspective on topics of critical importance to the health care industry today.

12. Champlin L. (1991). 'Eldercare' goal: integrate health, social needs. Geriatrics, 46(8):67.

A subtle revolution in health care for the elderly may be under way in the U.S. Administration on Aging (AoA). For the first time, AoA public policy makers are officially viewing housing, transportation, personal finances, and the full range of social issues as part of an elderly person's health care needs. This movement is being called the "National Eldercare Campaign." The recommendation from AoA proposes developing thirteen institutes, each of which will receive grants to identify needs and provide technical assistance, information, and other specific services. Examples of institutes are: long-term care, elder abuse, health promotion, and income security.

13. Dunkle R. E., Wykle M. L. (1988). Decision Making in Long-Term Care. New York: Springer Publishing Company.

Four major sections are included in this valuable resource book: Health Care Policy and Ethical Issues, Psychosocial Perspectives, Legal Parameters, and Cost. The chapter "The Family, the Elderly, and Long-Term Care" relates directly to home care and the need for more help of all kinds for caregivers who are generally spouses and adult children of older parents. Comprehensive overview of long-term care.

14. Dychtwald E., Zitter M., Levison J. (1990). New Directions for Eldercare Services. New York: McGraw-Hill.

The rapid growth in the number of elderly people in the U.S. is causing acute strains in our ability to provide care at all levels. The authors of this helpful book suggest that caregiver persons might best be organized by means of a stratified system, from assistance with changes in life style and in access to services such as transportation at the lower level, through health promotion and wellness programs, ambulatory care of acute and chronic problems, and care in the later years as the individual becomes more frail and disabled, which may require hospital or nursing home care. This continuum would permit better organization and allocation of scarce resources and, at the same time, provide managed care for optimal wellness at all stages of growing old.

15. Ferrini A. F., Ferrini R. L. (1989). Health in the Later Years. Dubuque, IA: William C. Brown Publishers.

A section within the chapter on "Long-Term Care" focuses on the history, services, benefits, and limitations of home health care. Figures from 1986 that show utilization of home care services indicate that this rate is quite low, primarily because of limited availability and accessibility. This book is recommended for health care providers and general readers.

16. Gubrium J. F., Sankar A. (1991). The Home Care Experience. Newbury Park, CA: Sage Focus Editions, Volume 119.

This book focuses on the social context of the home and how caregiving in the home can change the setting. Commonly held assumptions regarding home care and caregiving are discussed. Health care professionals will find this information helpful in gaining greater insight into the home care experience so that they can become more effective in their relationships with elderly clients and their families.

17. Halmandaris V. J. (1991). Home care: The cornerstone of long-term care for elderly Americans. Caring, 10(5):30-35.

This author states that the only solution to this country's devastating long-term care problems among the elderly is the enactment of a federally funded program under which the disabled and chronically ill individuals are eligible for a broad range of home-based services, regardless of their ability to pay. Without federal support, the financial burden falls wholly on the elderly person and the family. Home care, while perhaps not more cost-effective or efficient than institutional care, helps to keep families together and to preserve patients' dignity and independence.

18. Harper M. S. (1989). Behavioral, social, and mental health aspects of home care for older Americans.

<u>Home Health Care Services Quarterly</u>, <u>9</u>(4):61-123.

This is an important information sourcebook for educators, researchers, and health care professionals who are concerned with the health care provided to the elderly. Useful insights are discussed regarding evaluation outcomes of the various kinds of care and support that have been available to patients and their caregivers.

19. Hendrickson M. C. (ed.) (1986). <u>The Role of the Church in Aging</u>. Binghamton, NY: Haworth Press.

Three volumes are included in this series. Volume 1 provides implications for policy and action. Volume 2 describes implications for practice and service. Volume 3 highlights programs and services for the elderly. The multiplicity of topics presented in this series reflects the diversity of a growing aging population.

20. <u>Home Health Care</u> (1987). Report of a Conference on Issues, Trends, and Strategies. Sponsored by the Division of Nursing, Bureau of Health Professions, Health Resources and Services Administration, Department of Health and Human Services. (Accession # HRP-0907168, NTIS, Springfield, VA).

This conference explored the impact of a rapidly changing health care delivery system on the provision of quality home health care. Current issues and trends are identified and strategies were developed to ensure quality home health nursing care in the future.

21. Iverson L. H., Owens S. et al (1988). <u>Inter-Study's Long-Term Expansion Program: Issues Papers</u>. Excelsior, MN: Inter-Study Center for Aging and Long-Term Care.

This collection provides overviews of topics that are issues in long-term care. Concise information is presented by experts in the field in graphic and summary form that allows the complex data to be read easily. A resource for developing both undergraduate and graduate courses on long-term and home health care.

22. Justice D. (1990). State community-based care systems. Generations:45-48, spring.

How states have tried to strike a balance between flexibility and cost control of statewide community-based care systems is described in this article. The need for a federal long-term care policy is stressed to assure that all persons have access to needed care. The policy will have to provide significant discretion to states in order to reflect differences across the country in patterns of human services delivery and to capitalize on the infrastructure already in place.

23. Kovar M. G., Feinleib M. (1991). Older Americans present a double challenge: Preventing disability and providing care. Amer J Publ Health, 81 (3):287-88.

This editorial proposes that these two areas should be major goals of public health. While people are living longer (in 1987, two years longer than in 1978-81), there is no evidence that the length of disability-free life has increased at all. Data indicate that the number of years older persons are disabled has increased. The major plea is the need to increase data about chronic diseases and disability among the elderly as a basis for future planning toward providing adequate health care services.

24. McConnell S. (1990). Who really cares about long-term care? Generations:15-18, spring.

This article is a review of national opinion surveys regarding who is really concerned about long-term care in this country. Included in the review are issues related to the importance of long-term care, priorities in terms of public opinion, spending priorities, government vs private insurance responsibility, the willingness to pay taxes, and the type of program preferred. Noted in this report is that the great importance of long-term care rests in the fact that this issue touches the lives of so many American families in unique and critical ways.

25. Medalie J. H. (1989). The elderly and their families. In Clinical Aspects of Aging, 3rd ed. W. Reichel (ed.) Baltimore: Williams and Wilkins: 477-86.

The changing roles and relationships among family members are discussed in this chapter, relative to increasing age of older members. Factors that affect roles and relationships include changes in physical and mental health, financial assets and liabilities, burden on caregivers, housing and environment, decision making with respect to care and placement of older persons, individual and family needs, level of activities, and others. Family members, social workers, and care providers will find the case studies useful.

26. Monk R. S. (1990). Health Care of the Aged: Needs, Policies and Services. Binghamton, NY: Haworth Press.

Scholars and practitioners in gerontology address current and major issues of health care for older persons: policies, economics, levels of care, models of service delivery, and impact of the rapid increase in the number of older persons. Recommended for policy planners, administrators of home care services, and care providers.

27. Ory M. G., Duncker A. P. (1991). In-Home Health Care for Older People. Newbury Park, CA: Sage Publications.

This book focuses on different models for providing in-home care for the elderly and meeting the needs of caregivers. The various models are examined for effectiveness, efficiency, quality assurance, and coordination. Also addressed is the extent to which the Federal government should be involved in assuring that the needs of the elderly and their caregivers are met. Recommended for policy planners, administrators of home care agencies, and care providers.

28. Petersen M.D., White D. L. (eds.) (1989). Health Care of the Elderly: An Information Sourcebook. Newbury Park, CA: Sage Publications.

Sections and chapter titles include Substantive and Methodological Considerations: Critical issues, Literature review; Organization and Delivery of Care: Home and community care, Predictors and factors in nursing home and home care use, Case management, and Nursing home case-mix measurement; Social Support Programs: Gender, marital status, and childlessness in terms of availability of informal assistance, Shared housing, Respite services for family caregivers; Critical Care Issues and Physician Education: Prevention of osteoporosis, Iatrogenic illness, Comprehensive assessment, and Geriatrics-related continuing medical education.

29. Saucier K. A. (ed.) (1991). Perspectives in Family and Community Health. St Louis: Mosby:159-164.

This chapter addresses home care nursing practice, changing models of practice, lack of supportive and preventive care, the history of financing home care, and home care strategies for a new frontier. This book helps to place home care within the framework of public health and focuses on current issues and trends. Health care providers and caregivers will find this useful for background information and as a reference.

30. Serow W. J., Sly D. F., Wrigley J. M. (1990). Population Aging in the United States. Westport, CT: Greenwood Press.

This comprehensive book provides factual and statistical information about aging in America since 1900. A multitude of aspects of aging are presented on socioeconomic status, housing, health care needs, aging in place, and prevention of institutionalization. A useful reference for researchers, health professionals, and policy planners.

31. Sherman S. R., Newman E. S. (1988). Foster Families for Adults: A Community Alternative in Long-Term Care. New York: Columbia University Press.

The authors highlight a service option not well recognized as a treatment choice for the dependent older person. They provide the historical development of foster family care and a review of research on three adult populations in foster family care. Several variables were examined: the nature of family life in foster family care, the relationship between residents and the communities in which they live, and the roles of client, care provider, and agency. Students, faculty, policy planners and researchers will find this resource a useful addition to their library.

32. Spiegel A. D. (1983). Home Health Care. Owings Mills, MD: National Health Publishing.

This comprehensive study of home health care touches on many relevant issues: history of homecare, homemakers and home health aides, needs assessment for both individuals and population groups, diseases and conditions commonly found in people receiving home health care, planning and delivery of services, policy issues, financing, and others. A major resource is the comprehensive bibliographic citations at the end of chapters. Recommended as a basic source of information, much of which is useful almost ten years later.

33. Staebler R. (1991). Home based care: Easing the aging process. Caring, 10(5):1.

This editorial provides added impetus to the trend toward home care that is occurring across the country. The purposes of this publication are to describe the benefits of home care to policymakers and health care providers, to provide the latest information to assist health care workers in their profession, and to demonstrate to society that just because a person is sick, old, or disabled does not mean that they can no longer be useful and productive.

34. Stewart J. E. (1979). Home Health Care. St Louis: Mosby.

This book presents an overview of home care, types of agencies, basic services provided, related essential services, financing home care, continuity of care, and current trends. Although the content is now somewhat dated, there is much useful information that can be extrapolated to today's home health care system.

35. The Urban Institute (1991). A Project Report: The Needs of the Elderly in the 21st Century. Washington, DC: Policy Information Center.

This report predicts a surge in the number of elderly living alone who will exert additional pressure for expanded long-term care, home care, and social and housing services. The experts note that while many of the factors driving the need for elderly care are exogenous, many are within our power to influence. The focus is on reducing the incidence of disability, reforming the health care delivery system, and developing new financing mechanisms to make the purchase of needed services affordable for all who need them.

36. U.S. Department of Commerce, Bureau of Census, Current Population Reports, Special Studies, Series P-23, No. 153 (1990). America's Centenarians: Data from the 1980 Census. Washington, DC: Government Printing Office.

This report presents a profile of centenarians in this country, based on 1980 census data. The implications regarding the specific needs of this increasingly elderly population are evident. The differences between white and minorities are highlighted and the impact on home health care services is clear. All health care professionals need to be aware of these demographic changes and their potential influence for future health care planning and delivery in all settings, particularly in home health care.

37. Wasik B. H., Bryant D. M., Lyons C. M. (1990). Home Visiting: Procedures for Helping Families. Newbury Park, CA: Sage Publications.

Administrators, researchers, and students will find this volume to be a valuable reference book in their work with the elderly in the home. Important issues regarding home-visitation methods are discussed. How to carry out family support programs successfully in the home setting is highlighted.

2

Factors Affecting Home Care

A. Policy Issues:

38. Anderson J. M. (1990). Home care management in chronic illness and the self-care movement: An analysis of ideologies and economic processes influencing policy decisions. Adv Nurs Sci, 12 (2):71-83.

With the growth of home care and self-care emphasis come related economic and sociopolitical factors such as cost of care which should be assessed from both humanistic and economic perspectives. This thought-provoking article presents aspects of the issues cited with a view toward making changes in the amount of insurance coverage for costs related to home care.

39. Blumenthal D., Rizzo J.A. (1991). Who cares for uninsured patients? A study of physicians and their patients who lack health insurance. Medical Care, 29(6):502-520.

Physician involvement with uninsured patients is a topic of increasing policy interest. In the past, data limitations have hindered analysis of factors influencing physician contact with uninsured patients. This article attempts to bridge this gap in the health services literature. While definitive evidence that people without coverage face serious access problems is not provided, such a conclusion is certainly consistent with the findings in this study. The expectation is that this issue will continue to be an agenda item for policy planners.

40. Callahan D. (1989). Old age and new policy. JAMA, 261 (6):905-906.

Faced with the increasing deficits in the present Medicare program, this author concludes that we must rethink our goals for health in old age and reduce our insatiable appetite for longer life regardless of expense. The failure of efforts to control costs through efficiency measures has forced elderly persons to forgo optimal long-term or home care. The author points out that the public continues to expect more and better health care, with no corresponding inclination to pay the price. He recommends that entitlement progams must shift from short-term, critical care medicine for the elderly to the provision of care that improves the quality of everyday life, while not extending life by heroic efforts and the use of high tech methods.

41. Cottingham P. H., Ellwood D. T. (1989). Welfare Policy for the 1990s. Cambridge, MA: Harvard University Press.

This book presents three schools of thought regarding welfare reform. The approaches are to fix the current welfare system by targeting services more effectively, imposing new obligations, or altering case management methods, to rely on such nonwelfare supports as expanded health subsidies outside the welfare system, child care tax credits, or wage subsidies, and to reform macro-economic policies in several areas.

42. de Lissovoy G., Feustle J.A. (1991). Advanced home health care. Health Policy, 17:227-242.

This article reviews the evolution of home health care and the transition from patient-centered care to device-based care, with the former generally referred to as low-tech when providers described patients in terms of specific diseases and the latter focusing on therapeutic modalities: dialysis, infusion therapy, cardiac monitoring, etc. The authors state that this differentiation between low-tech and high-tech is artificial and does not facilitate home care planning or policy formulation. This comprehensive and authoritative article is highly recommended for policy planners and all who are engaged in any aspect of home care.

43. Fogel B. S., Furino A., Gottlieb, G. L. (1990). Mental Health Policy for Elder Americans: Protecting Minds at Risk. Washington, DC: American Psychiatric Association Press.

This is a well-researched and well-organized book on the complexities of state, federal, and private-sector policies regarding mental health care for elderly Americans. Noted experts review the clinical and epidemiological dimensions of mental illness, relate them to current financing and delivery programs, and offer a research and action agenda designed to make neuropsychiatric care more accessible and affordable for older persons.

44. General Accounting Office (1982). Elderly Should Benefit from Expanded Home Health Care but Increasing These Services Will Not Insure Cost Reductions. Washington, DC: Policy Information Center, PIC ID# 1528.

When expanded home health care services were offered to chronically ill elderly, client satisfaction and increased longevity resulted. The GAO recommended that more research is needed on the effects of expanded services for those elderly at risk for institutionalization, on hospital admission and recidivism rates, and on lengths of stay. The policy issue considered critical by this study was how to organize services for maximum effectiveness and efficiency.

45. Home Health Care: Present and Future Options. (1986). ERIC #ED-272817.

This document is the text of the Congressional hearings relative to present and future policies on home health care for the aged. One of the major issues discussed is the reliance on institutional care and the amount of Medicare and Medicaid money spent on nursing home services.

46. Lamy P. P. (1991). New approaches to old problems. Elder Care News, 7(2).

This editorial describes the FDA's proposal to require that information about the effects of prescription drugs be included on the labels. This requirement is particularly important for drugs commonly prescribed for the elderly. The announcement follows closely the recent notice on testing of drugs in the elderly, which has not been previously required by the FDA. These requirements are linked to the Health Objectives of the Nation for the Year 2000, and Healthy People 2000, the Surgeon General's reports to the nation.

47. Levenson S. A. (1989). Competence issues and adult protective services for the elderly. In Clinical Aspects of Aging, 3rd ed. W. Reichel (ed.). Baltimore: Williams and Wilkins: 504-509.

This chapter deals with competence of the elderly as this relates to the laws and regulations in place for five areas: those things society expects of persons permitted to live and function independently and autonomously in the community; the means of determining those who cannot meet such standards; the procedures for dealing with those who do not or cannot meet the standards; the legal and professional duties of those who deal with those individuals; and the nature and authority of the available resources and services for those who either cannot function appropriately or who can do so only with assistance. Recommended for policy planners, practitioners, lawyers, and families.

48. Lewin M. E., Sullivan S. (1989). The Care of Tomorrow's Elderly. Washington, DC: American Enterprise Institute for Public Policy Research.

The content of this paper addresses primarily policy issues related to health care financing, with chapters by contributors focusing on various aspects: insurance, the plight of many older persons, and a critique of the current system--Medicaid and Medicare--with a view toward possible changes. Coverage for home care under Medicare and Medicaid is quite limited and is tied to services ordered by physicians for those on a clear path to recovery, which the authors consider a major flaw. The rates of increased costs of home care reflect both the rising costs of care and, more important, the change in the services provided, with users receiving more of each kind of service.

49. Meiners M. R. (1982). Long-Term Care Insurance: Premium Estimates for Prototype Policies. Washington, DC: Policy Information Center, PIC ID# 1808.

The long-term care needs of the elderly have pressured the Medicaid and Medicare system to the extent that private insurance is being examined as an alternative strategy for reimbursement. This report provides premium estimates for prototype long-term care insurance policies as a basis for determining the feasibility of using private insurance to pay for care of the elderly in all settings. Administrators, and financial and policy planners will find this resource useful, although somewhat dated.

50. Moody H. R. (1988). Abundance of Life: Human Development Policies for an Aging Society. New York: Columbia University Press.

The question posed in this book is: How will public policy respond to the ever-growing group of older adults who are better educated and in better health than ever before. One solution is to mobilize this expanding group into a national resource rather than continue to view it as a burgeoning problem. One way to promote this concept is to use public action to increase the capacity for social contribution of older persons through work programs as continuing education, mutual help, voluntary action, and increased participation.

51. Rochefort D. A. (ed.) (1989). Handbook on Mental

<u>Health Policy in the United States</u>. Westport, CT: Greenwood Press.

This useful resource addresses public mental health policy in the U.S. Content examines mental health problems, policies, programs, and services, beginning with an overview of the policy arena and a review of psychiatric epidemiological methodology. A concise history of mental health policy from the seventeenth century is included. Analysis of needs assessment and strategic planning are discussed. The book ends with an essay about the future agenda for mental health policy.

52. Roland M. E., Schmidt R. M. (1989). The AIDS challenge to the regulation of experimental drugs. <u>Generations</u>:40-44, fall.

AIDS, health care, and the issues of access to experimental treatments are discussed in the context of implications for policy decisions and policies in place. Few research studies have been done about drug therapy in the elderly, in whom drug treatment is complicated by many factors. Policy changes are discussed regarding AIDS and drug review and approval procedures, which may place AIDS activists in conflict with researchers and policy makers. Administrators, policy planners, and health professionals need to be informed about current activities in order to fill the role of patient advocate.

53. Sultz H. (1991). Health policy: If you don't know where you're going, any road will take you. <u>Amer J Publ Health</u>, <u>81</u>(1):118-120.

Harry Sultz has for many years been actively engaged in research relating to health and health policy. In this article, he decries the lack of policy to support a health care delivery system that has no articulated purpose or some common vision that can be expressed as policy. Such a policy is needed to address difficult issues, to rid the present system of ambiguity of purpose, of ambivalence towards performance standards, conflicts of principles, and contradictions of goals.

He suggests that the American Public Health Association has among its members leaders of the character and quality required to plan, develop, and implement needed policies to direct changes in the health care system over the next few decades, and it is time we got on with it.

54. Weissert W. G. (1991). A new policy agenda for home care. Health Affairs, 10(2):67-77.

Research over 30 years and current estimates show that home care is neither cost-effective nor efficacious in improving long term health status. Although home care is the preferred choice to enable the elderly to live independently in their own homes, budget constraints are restricting public expenditures for these services. The author proposes strategies to increase efficiency and cost-effectivness of home care, which include improved screening, reducing hospital use, and increased use of managed care to set priorities, develop criteria, and make rationing choices among home care patients. Recommended for administrators and policy planners.

B. Costs:

55. Ansak M. L. (1990). The On Lok Model: Consolidating care and financing. Generations:773-74, spring.

The six principles that underlie the On Lok Model of care for very frail elderly in the San Francisco area are described in this article. Since 1983, On Lok has used a waiver system of payment, allowing for prospective monthly payments from Medicare, Medicaid, and individuals (based on the individual's entitlement) to meet all the health and health-related needs of its more than 300 very elderly and frail participants. The Pace Project, a replication of the On Lok Model around the country, is also described.

56. Atkins L. G. (1990). The politics of financing long-term care. Generations:19-22.

The complexities of enacting comprehensive financing of long-term care are discussed in light of Congress' repeal and attempted reform of the Medicare Catastrophic Coverage Act of 1988. Included in the discussion are lessons learned from catastrophic coverage, its unpopularity, and the need for political leadership.

57. Boyd B. (1990). LTC insurance: It's your choice. Generations:23-27, spring.

An insurance executive looks at options for LTC insurance from the private sector. The role of the insurance industry is continued growth of private long-term care insurance. The necessity of clearly describing benefit options and costs of public and private programs so that people can make appropriate choices is highlighted.

58. Brown F. (1983). Public Programs Financing Long-Term Care. Washington, DC: Policy Information Center, ID# 2283.2

This report contains comprehensive descriptions of the programs that support the elderly or disabled in our country's long-term care system. Programs described include those covered under the Older Americans Act, Title XX, long-term care programs operated by the Veterans Administration, and various other housing programs for these populations. Details are provided for each state in terms of utilization and variations in public financing across states. Findings from this report would be particularly useful for researchers.

59. Catalano D. J. (1989). Daily money management and protective services. Generations:74-75, fall.

This article provides a description of an integration of AIDS and aging service delivery. A discussion focuses on the need for staff in the formal support system to be well versed in money management and protection services for the elderly, since caregivers often become overwhelmed by their multiple responsibilities and must turn to professionals for help in these areas. Entrepreneurial practitioners have integrated these skills into their case management activities. Recommended for families, caregivers, and financial advisors.

60. Fama T., Kennell D. L. (1990). Should we worry about induced demand for long-term care services? Generations:37-41, spring.

Induced demand is defined as the effect of insurance upon demand for long-term care services. Financing of long-term care is at the center of the debate for reform. Potential concerns about the impact of proposed financing changes on service are discussed and include a section on induced demand for home care. Various studies are presented and, because of their shortcomings, the authors recommend that a carefully designed experimental study could test more directly whether price affects demand as is currently thought.

61. Friedland R. B. (1990). Facing the Costs of Long-Term Care: An EBRI-ERF Policy Study. Washington, DC: Employee Benefit Research Institute.

The content of this valuable book includes detailed documentation of existing data related to income, medical care expenditures and current methods of financing, a discussion of policy options for financing long-term care, and conclusions about the part that both public and private insurance play in financing long-term care. Evident in the data is the continuing need for the kind of careful analysis and data collection that are represented in this work.

62. General Accounting Office (1990). In-Home Services for the Elderly: Cost Sharing Expands Range of Services Provided and Populations Served. Washington, DC: Policy Information Center, ID# 3567.

Approaches to cost-sharing for in-home services for the elderly are examined in detail. Major topics included are 1) the option to charge fees for Older Americans Act program services provided to elderly clients who have the ability to pay, 2) the extent to which states use cost-sharing, 3) the types of services being cost-shared, 4) types of fee schedules used, 5) the benefits and disadvantages of cost-sharing, and 6) the characteristics of clients participating in these cost-sharing programs. Recommended for home care agency administrators and policy planners.

63. General Accounting Office (1990). Medicare: Need to Strengthen Home Health Care Payment Controls and Address Unmet Needs. Washington, DC: Policy Information Center, ID# 2904.

Three broad topics are covered in this report on Medicare Home Health programs: 1) effectiveness of program controls, 2) characteristics of users, and 3) extent of unmet home care needs reported by a sample of chronically ill elderly. The study concluded that further analysis was needed to determine why Medicare beneficiaries were unable to receive all the help they needed or why some types of users were most likely to have unmet needs or to receive uncovered services. This report is a source of information about Medicare reimbursement levels for administrators of home health care agencies.

64. Harrington C., Newcomer R. J. (1990). Social health maintenance organizations. Generations:40-54, spring.

Results of the Health Care Financing Administration's support of demonstration projects that developed innovative models for financing and delivering long-term care services to frail elderly are described in this article. The Social Health Maintenance Organization model (SHMO), established at Brandeis University, is the chief focus for the discussion. Many problems were encountered but the overall strategy is considered a unique approach to providing a complete range of acute and long-term care benefits to be effective in keeping chronic care utilization and costs within the SHMO budget targets.

65. Hays A. M. (1989). Paying for long-term care.

Geriatric Nurs, 10(1):20-21.

This short piece provides a brief review of trends in numbers of older persons and the costs of all types of long-term care.

66. Hellman, S., Hellman, L. H. (1991). Medicare and Medigap: A Guide to Retirement Health Insurance. Newbury Park, CA: Sage Publications.

This resource book provides a clear explanation of Medicare benefits and Medigap provisions suitable for professionals, beneficiaries, and their caregivers. Clear, comprehensive information describes retirement issues and simplifies the filing of claims and organzation of medical papers, forms, and other materials for Medicare recipients.

67. Hoyer R. G. (1991). Public programs for the elderly: Can we afford them? Caring, 10(5):4-13.

The author states that some people believe that the U.S. is spending more on Social Security and Medicare than it can afford, and argues that these programs should be curtailed. However, the author refutes these claims and says that wealthy senior citizens are the exception, not the rule; most elderly persons have limited private funds. Further, the author contends that recent articles about intergenerational conflicts are overstating that issue, which he considers to be minor in nature. Current needs of families, particularly with respect to children, could have long-range repercussions for the future of the country. Curtailing those programs that are meeting these needs is not the solution.

68. Kane N. M. (1989). The home care crisis of the nineties. Gerontologist, 29(1):24-31.

This article describes trends found in publicly owned, for-profit custodial home care agencies, and recommends needed changes in the financing of home care. Restrictive public payments and limited private insurance coverage were seen as major barriers for providers and, thus, for those needing home care services. Included is a well thought out analysis of the current status and projected problems in financing home care in the decades ahead. Recommended for administrators, and financial and policy planners.

69. Liu K. (1990). Recent changes in the Medicare skilled nursing facility benefit. Generations:75-76, spring.

This article enlightens the reader on the historical development of Medicare coverage for skilled nursing facility care coverage between 1987 and 1989, during which an increase occurred that far surpassed official projections. New policies developed during April 1988 are described and generally acknowledge the shift in emphasis from post-acute and self-limiting conditions to serious conditions requiring skilled nursing care. Information included is important for all health care professionals caring for the elderly to know. Congress will continue deliberations regarding future reforms in health care coverage issues.

70. Longman P. (1987). Born to Pay: The New Politics of Aging in America. Boston: Houghton Mifflin.

The subject of this book is generational differences between the large group of elderly who are retired and living on pensions, and their children who are members of the Baby Boom years, now in their forties, who are required to make up the deficit between retirement incomes and living expenses for their aging parents. The problem addressed is that of distribution of justice between these two groups. Should the costs of health care, retirement, and insurance fall upon the shoulders of the younger generation? Recommended for families, caregivers, providers, and policy planners.

71. Mahoney K. J. (1990). The Connecticut partnership for long-term care. Generations:71-72, spring.

The development of an economical, feasible, and mutually beneficial model using public and private funds cooperatively to finance long-term care for the elderly in the state of Connecticut is described as one of the state's major accomplishments. Some of the experiences in the process have relevance regarding a national approach to financing long-term care for the elderly. Health care providers need to be informed about such activities if they are to play a vital role in policy planning and developing the best possible means of caring for this population.

72. Medicare and the American Health Care System: Report to Congress (1991). Washington, DC: Prospective Payment Assessment Commission.

This comprehensive report includes all aspects of Medicare and Medicaid expenditures, benefits, and projections regarding the health care system, insurance coverage, access to care, and reforms being considered in all these and other areas. This report provides a rich source of information for policy planners, health care administrators and professionals, and those in private and public health insurance.

73. Meiners M. R., McKay H. L. (1990). Private vs. social long-term care insurance: Beware the comparison. Generations:32-36, spring.

The feasibility of making adjustments to the Medicaid program in order to improve our long-term care system is discussed in this article. Partnership programs supported by the Robert Wood Johnson Foundation in various states are described and the interventions being explored by the states are outlined. The experience of these states in creating and administering partnership financing programs is seen as a basis for further reform to the current system or for the creation of a national insurance system.

74. Mogey J. (ed.) (1990). Aiding and Aging: The Coming Crisis in Support for the Elderly by Kin and State. Westport, CT: Greenwood Press.

This collection of essays and survey analyses explores

the way aging affects society. The U.S. and Hungary--two quite different systems--are compared with respect to the relationship between social support and aging. Support derives from formal and informal systems; however, support from formal systems was preferred in both countries. The focus is maintained on the need to encourage persistence of the kinship system and continuance of public programs to maintain the elderly in their homes.

75. Myles J. (1989). Old Age in the Welfare State: The Political Economy of Public Pensions. Lawrence: University Press of Kansas.

In the last five years, there has been a continuing policy debate about income security for the elderly. Often, discussions focus on the burden on working-age adults who are children of the elderly. The author's major premise is that the economic well-being of the elderly in the advanced capitalist democracies is the outcome of a political process, a premise that is relevant to the current debate about the future of our public pension system - social security. Highly informative content on many aspects of public pensions in Western countries.

76. Nicoll L. H., Niman N. B. (1991). Deficit reduction and healthcare expenditures: a macroeconomic perspective. J Nurs Admin, 21(6):35-39.

The federal budget deficit is a serious problem facing the U.S. economy, and reductions in the deficit have been mandated by Congress. The authors present the potential direct and indirect effects of such reductions on the healthcare system. Strategies for nurse executives to deal with pressures that arise from a changing economic environment are discussed.

77. Office of Audit (1990). Follow-Up Review: Medicare Need to Strengthen Home Health Care Payment Controls and Address Unmet Needs. Washington, DC: Policy Information Center, ID# 2904.1.

This audit report determined whether actions taken by the Health Care Financing Administration resolved problems noted in the above-referenced GAO Report. Conclusions reached were: 1) home health coverage criteria have been clarified and HCFA is in the process of implementing prepayment utilization screens for home health services, 2) statistical sampling methods in postpayment reviews of home health agencies have not been implemented, and 3) the Contractor Performance Evaluation Program's responsibilities have been expanded to include the assessment of the accuracy of intermediary home health coverage determinations and to further study factors contributing to unmet needs for home care assistance.

78. Pegels C. C. (1988). Health Care and the Older Citizen: Economic, Demographic, and Financial Aspects. Rockville, MD: Aspen Publishers, Inc.

This informative book provides an analysis of these and other factors affecting health care and health care delivery. A separate chapter addresses home health care objectives, programs, and services. A division of services has occurred with distinct classifications of types of services available. These classifications, which are frequently quite separate, are prevention, support, and therapeutic. Provider organizations and individuals, however, should keep these categories in mind and try to develop bridges between and among them. This bridging will inevitably result in improved and more comprehensive care.

79. The Pepper Report: Blueprint for long-term care coverage (1990). Caring, 10(2):32-34.

This article is an excerpt from the Pepper Commission Report, A Call For Action, Chapter 4. Washington, DC: Government Printing Office. The Commission stated that all Americans should have the security of knowing that if the need for long-term care should arise--for themselves, their parents or their children--they would have a national long-term care system in place to turn to for help. Coverage should be affordable for all, provide for personal choice of care and setting, assure quality care, and provide for consumer protection.

80. Polich C. L., Iverson L. H. et al (1988). Inter-Study's Long-Term Care Expansion Program: A Proposal for Reform. Excelsior, MN: Inter-Study Center for Aging and Long-Term Care.

This is the first of a two-volume series whose intent is to examine the financing system for long-term care of the elderly and develop a proposal for reform. The group proposed a social insurance approach which would create a Medicare Part C by combining all long-term care services currently funded by Medicare and Medicaid. This is viewed as the most cost-effective approach to long-term care insurance in the U.S. Must reading for all concerned with long-term care financing.

81. Rivlin A. M., Wiener J. M. (1988). Caring for the Disabled Elderly: Who Will Pay? Washington, DC: The Brookings Institution.

Content about home health care focuses on the impact of amount, type, and quality of services as determined by economic conditions. Various methods for financing long term care are addressed, in both private and public sectors. Suggestions are offered for future funding for home care services into the next century. Recommended for administrators and health finance policy planners.

82. Schneider E. L., Guralnik J. M. (1990). The aging of America: Impact on health care costs. JAMA, 263(17):-2335-2340.

A large number of Americans are surviving into their 80s and 90s. This fastest growing age group of the "oldest old" (those aged 85 years and older) will have a substantial impact on health care costs in the coming decades. Using current U.S. Census Bureau projections, the authors estimate that future costs for Medicare, nursing homes, and home care will rise sharply, and that costs for specific conditions such as dementia and hip fractures will compound the financial situation. Cost containment measures alone will not be sufficient to slow health care costs for the elderly. The authors recommend increased funding for biomedical research to improve our ability to prevent or cure diseases and disabilities associated with aging.

83. Schwartberg J. G., Stein-Hulin J. (1991). Home health care: Surmounting the obstacles to Medicare coverage. Geriatrics, 46(4):28.

Specific terminology regarding home health services is critical to ensuring Medicare reimbursement for these services. Medicare coverage is based on a "disease" model. The physician must justify the "medical necessity" for home health care by listing all the medical diagnoses that affect the patient's ability to function. The patient must require skilled care in order to have the services covered by Medicare. Chronically ill patients who will never recover and whose condition(s) will deteriorate if services are not provided are the ideal candidates for home care benefits of skilled management and evaluation. Recommended for administrators of home health care agencies and policy planners.

84. Spence D. A., Hanley R. J. (1990). Public insurance options for financing long-term care. Generations:28-31, spring.

This article debates various public insurance options for financing long-term care and describes the advantages of public long-term care insurance. Current proposals under consideration are evaluated and conclusions are drawn. Thought-provoking article for all concerned with future coverage for long-term care; a must for health care providers.

85. University of Colorado Medical Center (1979). Cost Per Episode of Home Health Care. Washington, DC: Policy Information Center, ID# 0736.

In this study, cost is defined as including the total cost of skilled nursing, physical therapy, speech therapy, occupational therapy, social services, and home health aide visits in the home. Massachusetts and Pennsylvania were the selected sites. Significant differences were noted along with some similarities in the two sites. Findings, although somewhat dated, can be extrapolated to the present health care environment.

86. Vladeck B. C., Alfano G. J. (eds.) (1987). Medicare and Extended Care: Issues, Problems, and Prospects. Owings Mills, MD: National Health Publishing, a division of Rynd Communications.

Perspectives on extended care with selected case studies and financial issues are discussed. Different models of delivering extended care and rehabilitation to the elderly are presented. Some health care professionals need to be well informed about this area since they are frequently asked for guidance in determining if, when, and where extended care placement of their home care clients takes place.

87. Wiener J. M., Harris K. M. (1991). Regulation of private long-term care insurance. Caring, 10(5):36-42.

This article provides information about private long-term care insurance, and reports that there has been a significant improvement in the quality of this type of insurance policies over the past five years. However, as the market continues to expand and mature, national standards need to be assessed and, if necessary, strengthened to protect the insured. The authors believe that federal regulation is desirable because it is likely that, without a Federal mandate, some states will never adopt even minimally acceptable standards in this area.

88. Weissert W. G. (1990). Strategies for reducing home-care expenditures. Generations:42-44, spring.

This article focuses on looking at ways to make home care a cost-effective alternative to nursing home care. Reasonable goals for enhancing both the efficiency and the efficacy of home care are outlined. The importance and urgency of the problem are highlighted. A thought-provoking approach for educators, researchers, administrators, and health care providers.

C. Legal Issues:

89. Arnason S. (1990). The legal needs of the elderly: rights, wrongs, and remedies. Aging, no. 360:14-18.

According to the Commission on Legal Problems of the Elderly of the American Bar Association, many older Americans do not recognize that some of their problems are legal in nature. As a result, they do not seek help. If they are lucky, they talk to someone who is able to identify the nature of the problem and knows where to turn for assistance. If they are not so lucky, the problem can become a crisis. Poor elderly are probably the most vulnerable since they are more dependent on others for help. This comprehensive article provides valuable information to assist the elderly with problems that may have a legal basis.

90. Kennedy I. (1988). Treat Me Right: Essays in Medical Law and Ethics. Oxford: Clarendon Press.

Eighteen papers are gathered together in this one volume to illustrate the relationship between medical ethics and medical law. Fifteen of these papers have been previously published and three are new. Issues addressed include treatment of the terminally ill, organ donation, informed consent, and other ethical and legal problems that are of concern to interested health care professionals in all settings.

3

Care in the Home

A. Practice:

91. Abrams W. B., Berkow R. (eds.) (1990). The Merck Manual of Geriatrics. Rahway, NJ: Merck, Sharp & Dohme Laboratories.

This manual provides information of clinical relevance to all health care providers of the elderly. The contents are divided into five major areas that include a problem-oriented approach about nutrition problems, multiple approaches to assessment, prevention, diagnosis, and treatment therapies, medications, the risks and benefits of exercise, and legal-ethical issues. Reference tables regarding normal laboratory values and sample assessment instruments are included. A section on health care costs and insurance is helpful for practitioners and clients.

92. Anderson E. (1991). These foolish things: Reflections on older smokers and drinkers. Geriatrics, 46(2):71-74.

Many older persons may have health problems that are the result of years of smoking and drinking. Often, these people grew up in the era of the 1940s and 1950s when both behaviors were promoted by the movies, commercial advertising, and peer pressure. The question that this article addresses is: Is it too late now for these people to benefit by stopping smoking and drinking?

Studies show that many older persons can recover better functioning once these behaviors are eliminated, regardless of age or health status.

93. Baltimore M. N. (1990). Dementia Care: Patient, Family, and Community. Baltimore: The Johns Hopkins University Press.

An account of the holistic care needed by patients with dementias and their families is provided in this excellent resource. In three sections, the author describes patient care, working with families, and working with community groups. In the first section, information on designing the environment for cognitively impaired persons is especially helpful. Highly recommended for families, caregivers, and health care professionals who care for elderly persons with these kinds of conditions.

94. Belcher D. (1989). Prevention of osteoporosis in the elderly. In Health Care of the Elderly, Eds.: M. D. Petersen, D. L. White. Newbury Park, CA: Sage Publications, 413-450.

This chapter presents a review of the literature about prevention of osteoporosis. The focus is the effectiveness of interventions intended to prevent the condition, detection test used in screening for the condition, and the generalizability of findings from the studies cited. This condition is a major problem for and concern of elderly persons who are being cared for at home and their caregivers. Recommended for health professionals, nutritionists, exercise therapists, and interested others.

95. Bernstein L. H., Grieco A. J., Dete M. K. (eds.) (1987). Primary Care in the Home. Philadelphia: J. B. Lippincott Company.

This text describes home care as a process and the chapters cover the many situations and health problems that are managed in the home. The authors have an interdisciplinary focus and discuss the roles of health care providers, the importance of the home environment, and the partnerships that are needed between the providers and the family.

96. Bernstein L. H. (1991). An update on home intravenous antibiotic therapy. Geriatrics, 46(6):47-54.

Home intravenous antibiotic therapy (HIVAT) is a safe, effective, and cost-saving method to treat appropriately selected patients with bone, soft tissue, respiratory, genitourinary, and cardiac infections. The acceptability of HIVAT by both physicians and patients has been enhanced by new venous access devices and home IV therapy companies.

97. Bertram M. (1989). The use of landmarks. J Geront Nurs, 15(2):6-8.

The focus of this article is developing methods to maintain confused patients' orientation to date, time, place, and people, such as signs, arrows, calendars, and notes. This information is useful to caregivers and others working with the elderly.

98. Blass J. P. (1990). The report of the advisory panel on Alzheimer's disease, 1988-1989. Generations: 68-69, spring.

This is a summary of the first report on Alzheimer's disease issued by the Advisory Panel in 1989. Issues considered by this group and covered in the report include: 1) the need for biomedical research to find ways to prevent the disease, 2) the need for services which could not be considered apart from the general issues surrounding long-term care, and 3) the financing of care for these patients which were considered in concert with the more general problems around long-term care for the chronically ill. The panel's recommendations were considered as steps toward easing the burden of caregivers for these persons.

99. Brink T. L. (1986). Clinical Gerontology: A Guide to Assessment and Intervention. Binghamton, NY: Haworth Press.

The focus of this book is psychogeriatrics, addressing family therapy and mental health care of older persons through psychological management of problems common in the elderly. Recommended for practitioners as a resource guide.

100. Brody S. J., Pawlson L. G. (1990). Aging and Rehabilitation II: The State of the Practice. New York: Springer Publishing Company.

This excellent reference includes many aspects of disability. It covers such topics as independent living, specific disabling conditions, mental and emotional stress, legal problems prevalent among older persons, and social, environmental, and behavioral factors that affect recovery from or living with disability. Recommended for health professionals and caregivers.

101. Brown G. W., Harris T. O. (1989). Life Events and Illness. New York: The Guilford Press.

Contributors to this scientific work include experts from many disciplines - psychiatry, psychology, neurology, social policy, social sciences, community practice physicians, and others. Years of study and experiences with patients enabled these experts to produce this comprehensive book which explains the link between life events, and attitudes and illness. Specific conditions are discussed, e.g., multiple sclerosis. Highly recommended for health professionals in all disciplines.

102. Burgio L., Burgio K. (1986). Behavioral gerontology: Application of behavioral methods to the problems of older adults. Journal of Applied Behavior Analysis, 19(4):321-328.

This article addresses the role of behavior analysis in caring for elderly persons in the home and other settings. The authors stress the need for more research in many areas of behavioral gerontology, including the training of community caregivers. An excellent resource for researchers and practitioners in gerontology.

103. Carstensen L. L., Edelstein B. A. (1987). Handbook of Clinical Gerontology. New York: Pergamon Press.

This resource book offers broad coverage of a large number of clinical problems and treatment issues facing those who work with elderly persons. The 28 chapters are organized into five major areas: normal aging, psychiatric disorders, common medical problems, behavior problems, and social issues. The last section on social issues includes such topics as social support, politics and ethics, bereavement, housing needs and transitions, clinical issues for black elderly, and prevention of age-related problems. Highly recommended for all care providers for the elderly in all settings.

104. Condon E. H. (1989). Dementia and depression: A devastating pair. Geriatric Nurs, 10(1):26-27.

In patients with Alzheimer's disease, symptoms may mask an accompanying depression. Care providers and caregivers need to be aware of the differences so that underlying depression can be treated. This article presents distinguishing features of both, and ways to recognize and treat both conditions.

105. Cooper J. K. (1991). Alzheimer's disease: Answering questions commonly asked by patients' families. Geriatrics, 46:338-47.

When an elderly person is first diagnosed as having Alzheimer's disease, family members usually have a number of questions, ranging from concerns about genetic aspects of the condition to specific caregiving approaches. The patient and family caregiver need information, support, and assistance to deal with the multiple problems that result from this disease. This article discusses drug therapy, activities such as driving, legal issues such as power of attorney, and other topics related to progress of the disease. Recommended for lawyers, caregivers, and those involved in education about the disease.

106. De Luca H. F., Mazess R. (1990). Osteoporosis:

<u>Physiological Base, Assessment and Treatment</u>. New York: Elsevier Science Publishing Company.

This book comprises the proceedings of the Nineteenth Steenbock Symposium, June 5-8, 1989, at the University of Wisconsin, Madison. Content focuses on etiology, risks of fracture, methods of assessment, the role of estrogen, fluoride, Vitamin D, calcitonin, and exercise on bone integrity and health status.

107. Dunlap J., Manghelli D., Tolson R. (1990). Older problem drinkers: A community treatment continuum. <u>Aging</u>, no. 361:33-37.

In the last 10 to 15 years, there has been a growing awareness of the number of older persons who are alcoholics or who have problems related to alcohol consumption. Estimates of the number of elderly with this problem range from 2% to 19%. Modes of dealing with condition include prevention, outreach, intervention, detoxification services, protective environments, primary treatment, and continuing care. Project DARE (Drug and Alcohol Resources for the Elderly) provides information, educational materials, and technical assistance to organizations working with elders who have this problem. Contact: Project DARE, 3835 S.W. Kelly, Portland, OR 97201.

108. Enck R. E. (1991). Pain control in the ambulatory elderly. <u>Geriatrics</u>, <u>46</u>(3):49-60.

Pain control in the elderly, regardless of the cause, can be a major challenge in caring for these persons, especially in the home setting. Aging causes a decreased perception of pain and an increased sensitivity to opioid analgesics. This article presents an assessment of patients with pain and includes an objective instrument for evaluating pain from the perspective of both provider and patient. Content includes use and effects of various drugs, concerns about addiction, and the WHO Cancer Pain Relief Program. Highly recommended for health care professionals.

109. Gelfand B. (1991). <u>The Creative Practitioner</u>. Binghamton, NY: Haworth Press.

This text is particularly useful for health care practitioners in working with patients with multiple and complex problems. The author links creative thinking processes with problem solving in a thought-provoking and stimulating way. Helpful exercises are included that show how to access and utilize thinking processes.

110. Greene R. R. (1991). Supervision in social work with the aged and their families. <u>J Geront Soc Work</u>, <u>17</u>(1/2):139-144.

This paper focuses on the educational and supportive functions of the long-standing practice tradition of supervision in social work with the aged and their families. The author examines the way in which educational supervision extends clinicians' knowledge and deepens their perceptions, feelings, and self-understanding of geriatric care and practice. A case study is presented that illustrates job-related stress, ethical issues and values conflicts that can occur in working with the elderly and family members.

111. Grieco A. J. (1991). Physician's guide to managing home care of older patients. <u>Geriatrics</u>, <u>46</u>(5):49-60.

This broad conception of home care provides excellent guidance to professionals about coaching family members to give care and to assess their individual home/situation periodically to recognize and respond to changing needs of family members receiving care. The author emphasizes support and education to bridge the gap between care settings for those providing care. Recommended for practitioners and other health care professionals.

112. Haddad A. M. (1987). <u>High Tech Home Care: A Practical Guide</u>. Rockville, MD: Aspen Publishers, Inc.

Information about issues surrounding access, delivery, and liability of high tech services in the home is vital to administrators, practitioners, and owners of home care agencies. Discussion includes comprehensive home care, and the attendant competitive and regulatory forces that impact on it. Included are a Model Client Care Plan, a checklist for selecting a home care agency, and a section on legal issues encountered in the home care arena. The emphasis is on high touch to counteract the potential dehumanizing effects of high tech care. References at the end of each chapter provide extensive coverage of the broad scope of home care management, delivery, services, and the environments, both internal and external, in which they operate.

113. Handy C. M. (1988). Home care of patients with technically complex nursing needs. <u>Nurs Clin North Am</u>, <u>23</u>(2):315-325.

Patients requiring high tech nursing care are being discharged earlier from hospitals into the home setting. Home care agencies are facing increasing problems in meeting these complex care needs, with administrators having concerns about clinical competence of care providers, and the administrative, financial, and educational needs of the agency and its personnel. This author indicates that home care agency administrators find that the use of careful planning regarding use of personnel and distribution of available resources to address these concerns is the key to success in meeting the needs of both patients and personnel.

114. Harper M. (1991). <u>Management and Care of the Elderly</u>. Newbury Park, CA: Sage Publications.

This book focuses on the psychosocial, behavioral, and mental health needs of older adults. It provides direction for health professionals to assist caregivers in meeting these needs. Emphasis is placed on difficult cases such as Alzheimer's disease, racial-ethnic issues, and hostility in the elderly.

115. Hoffman N. B. (1991). Dehydration in the elderly: insidious and manageable. <u>Geriatrics</u>, <u>46</u>(6):45-48.

The elderly are at risk for dehydration, due to decreased thirst perception, decreased water intake, abnormal vasopressin responses to osmotic stimuli, and a predisposition to mild nephrogenic diabetes insipidus. Older persons, because of chronic physical or mental disabilities, may not be able to obtain sufficient water for themselves. Caregivers of elderly in the home need to be aware of this potential or actual problem.

116. Hogstel M. O., Kashka M. K. (1989). Staying healthy after 85, Geriatric Nurs, 10(1):16-18.

Factors deemed essential for good health in later years include exercise/work, sufficient sleep, a support system that includes firm philosophical or religious beliefs, adequate nutrition, no smoking, alcohol, or drugs, and a positive outlook on life. Recommended for caregivers and care providers of elderly clients, particularly in the home setting.

117. Jaffe K. B. (1989). Home health care and rehabilitation nursing. Nurs Clin North Am, 24(1):171-78.

Health care is increasingly being delivered in ambulatory and home settings. Hospitals have increased cost incentives to discharge patients more quickly, often resulting in older patients having greater home health care needs than was true in the past. Rehabilitation services in the home is an area of increased expansion, thus enabling the rehabilitation nurse to be an integral member of the interdisciplinary home care team.

118. Jarvik L. F., Wiseman E. J. (1991). A checklist for managing the dementia patient. Geriatrics, 46(5):31-40.

Primary care physicians and other care providers are seeing increasing numbers of elderly demented patients. This article presents the mnemonic FICS'M (Family, Intellectual Status, Continence, Sleep, and Mobility) checklist to help health professionals assess problems associated with dementing illnesses, and to initiate appropriate treatment with family or caregiver involvement. Interventions that take into account the physical, psychological, and social problems connected with dementia can susbstantially decrease morbidity.

119. Kane R. A., Kane R. L., Rubenstein L. Z. (1989). Comprehensive assessment of the elderly patient. In Health Care of the Elderly. Eds.: M. D. Petersen, D. L. White. Newbury Park, CA: Sage Publications, 475-519.

This chapter presents a review of the literature about geriatric assessment. The authors use a conceptual approach to the topic. The purpose is to answer research questions related to how the elements of comprehensive assessment have been conceptualized, and how the independent and dependent variables have been operationalized in the studies cited. Questions for researchers are raised regarding the analysis. In the summary are samples of instruments and techniques used in geriatric assessment which have implications for those responsible for home care of the elderly.

120. Kemp B., Brummel-Smith K., Ramsdell J. (eds.) (1991). Geriatric Rehabilitation. Boston: College Hill Press.

A practical handbook for health professionals who have concerns and care for the disabled elderly and their families. The book comprises five areas, including basic philosophical and geriatric rehabilitation concepts and theories, major disabling conditions, practical ways to improve functional abilities, rehabilitation of older persons with mental deficiencies and dementias, and the impact of technology on geriatric rehabilitation.

121. Knight B. (1986). Psychotherapy with Older Adults. Newbury Park, CA: Sage Publications.

This book provides an excellent discussion of therapy using case studies and summaries to clarify major points. Research findings are linked to practical experience which should be useful to psychiatrists, psychologists, social workers, and psychiatric nurses working with older adults in any setting.

122. Mazanec D. J. (1991). Conservative treatment of rheumatic disorders in the elderly. Geriatrics, 46(5):1-4.

Rheumatic problems are the most common cause of limited activity and disability in elderly patients. Those over 65 are particularly susceptible to adverse reactions to anti-rheumatic drug therapy, especially the nonsteroidal anti-inflammatory drugs (NSAIDs). Using an approach that emphasizes safety by employing nondrug therapy, conservative prescribing methods, and close monitoring of patients'reactions will enhance comfort and compliance level of activity in older persons.

123. Miller C. M. (1989). A past well remembered ... Geriatric Nurs, 10(1):28-29.

This short article stresses the importance of providing opportunities for older persons to reminisce and to talk about their memories, both for historical purposes and to allow older people to express their attitudes, opinions, and emotions through this medium, which can be remarkably therapeutic.

124. Murray F. E., Bliss C. M. (1991). Geriatric constipation: Brief update on a common problem. Geriatrics, 46(3):64-68.

Multiple factors can cause constipation in the elderly, and necessitate a search for the primary underlying cause by means of a comprehensive history and thorough physical examination. Some of the causes include irritable bowel syndrome, diverticulitis, neurologic conditions, and diet and environmental factors. Management should include adequate exercise and fluid intake, high fiber diet, regular bowel habits and, only as a last resort, drug therapy in the form of wetting and bulking agents.

125. National Institutes of Health Consensus Development Conference (1984). Osteoporosis. JAMA, 252(6):299-302.

Conclusions from the 1984 conference on osteoporosis conducted at the National Institutes of Health are presented. Osteoporosis is identified as the major underlying cause of bone fractures in postmenopausal women and older persons. The information derived from the conference needs to be disseminated more widely to health care professionals and to the general public.

126. National Institutes of Health Consensus Development Conference, July 6-8 (1987). Differential diagnosis of dementing disease. DHHS, PHS: <u>Office of Medical Applications Research</u>, <u>6</u>(11).

Dementia has its highest rate of occurrence in the population over the age of 75 years, the fastest growing age group in the country. Recent advances in science give hope that better methods of treatment will become available. Dementing diseases are described. Reversible and arrestable types of dementia are included. Topics covered by experts in the field were: 1) components of initial evaluation of dementia, 2) diagnostic tests to be used in the evaluation of dementia, and 3) priorities for future research on diagnostic methods. Valuable resource for all who work with the very old in any setting.

127. Palumbo M. V. (1990). Hearing access 2000: Increasing awareness of the hearing impaired. <u>Geront Nurs</u>, <u>16</u>(9):26-31.

Many older persons have decreased ability to hear. If others become more aware of this problem, the hearing impaired individual will be able to function at a higher level. Tips for communicating with a person with hearing loss are included. This is a valuable addition to care providers' information materials.

128. Papas A. S., Niessen L. C., and Chauncey H. H. (1991). <u>Geriatric Dentistry: Aging and Oral Health</u>. St. Louis: Mosby.

The range of topics in this outstanding text includes an overview on aging in America, physiology and biology of aging, effects of drug treatment, oral physiology, clinical care, assessment of the older adult, treatment planning, management of dental caries, specific dental problems commonly found in the elderly, management of problems, and preventive dentistry in the older patient. Useful resource for care providers, dentists, and others who work with the elderly in any setting.

129. Parzick J. A., Triebsch H. C. (eds.) (1991). Care of the Alzheimer's patient in the home setting. J Home Health Care Pract, 3(4):1-80.

This issue contains 11 articles by experts, relating to many aspects of caring for Alzheimer's patients. Topics include definition of the disease, therapy options, the caregiver's perspective, the role of social workers, nutrition, urinary incontinence, methods of communicating, dealing with the disoriented person, volunteers program, family decision making, and hands-on home care. This volume provides a wide range of information.

130. Porush J. G., Faubert P. F. (1991). Renal Disease in the Aged. Boston: Little, Brown.

Health care professionals need to keep informed about early symptoms, assessment and referral, and management of renal problems in the elderly. Content includes anatomy and physiology, disorders of water and salt metabolism, acid-base disorders, disorders of potassium, calcium, phosphorus and magnesium metabolism, primary glomerular disease, urolithiasis and obstructive uropathy, renal involvement in systemic disease, urinary infections, acute and chronic renal failure, hypertension, and renal vascular disease. Excellent resource.

131. Riggs B. L., Melton L. J. III (Eds.) (1988). Osteoporosis: Etiology, Diagnosis and Management. New York: Raven Press.

This book focuses on clinical aspects of the disease: physiological bases of bone, diagnostic methods, pathophysiology related to hormones and nutritional factors, and management. Many leading experts contributed to the excellence of this reference, recommended for care providers of the elderly in all settings.

132. Riley M. W., Ory M. G., Zablotsky D. (eds.) (1989). AIDS in an Aging Society: What We Need to Know. New York: Springer Publishing Company.

The knowledge, incidence, attitudes, and risk behaviors for AIDS in the elderly population are addressed in this volume. The authors provide information about what needs to be taught to the elderly and their caregivers to limit the epidemic's impact, and calls for more research in the social and behavioral sciences regarding the effects of this disease. This is a valuable resource for practitioners, researchers, and policy planners.

133. Riley M. W., Riley J. W., Jr. (1989). The quality of aging: Strategies for interventions. The Annals, 503.

This special issue presents evidence that we currently have the knowledge and capability to employ social interventions that can improve the quality of the aging process. However, related interventions have not been used as efficiently and effectively as they could be. While advances have occurred to foster individual psychological and physiological well-being, few interventions at the social level provide incentives or opportunities to enhance the aging process.

134. Snyder M., Brugge-Wiger P. et al (1991). Complex health problems: Clinically assessing self-management abilities. J Geront Nurs, 17(4):23-27.

The authors describe a new instrument recently developed to assess the self-management capabilities of elderly clients about to be discharged from acute care settings into the community. Adequate assessment of capabilities and deficits prior to discharge will help to ensure that appropriate interventions and supports can be provided. Results of a pilot study using the tool and implications for its incorporation into discharge planning are addressed.

135. Streckfus B. L. W., Bergers R. M. (1987). Infection control for caregivers of AIDS patients. NITA, 10(4):282-84.

Health care providers increasingly are facing the unique challenge of dealing with People With AIDS (PWAs). Practitioners in the home settings are confronted with even greater challenges to ensure that the level of sophisticated care necessary for these acutely ill individuals can be provided safely and effectively. Guidelines are included to assist caregivers to control the spread of the human immunodeficiency virus (HIV) to themselves and others who have direct contact with the AIDS patient. Recommended for health care professionals and others who work with PWAs.

136. Taira E. D., Maynard M., Madigan M. J. (eds.) (1989). Assessing the Driving Ability of the Elderly. Binghamton, NY: Haworth Press.

Techniques are presented to evaluate older drivers who have bcome physically, cognitively or otherwise impaired but who wish to continue to drive. This resource provides specific guidelines for working with older drivers. Recommended for caregivers and health care professionals.

137. Thompson M. P., Tollison J. W. (1990). Caring for the elderly. In Textbook of Family Practice, 4th Edition. Ed.: R. E. Rakel. Philadelphia: W. B. Saunders, 140-180.

This chapter provides an overview of older persons within the context of the social, political, and scientific milieux into which they were born, e.g., 1900, 1925, 1950. The authors address societal prejudices regarding the elderly, the most common causes of deterioration, a complete listing of physical changes that occur with aging, and treatment of health problems. This is a valuable resource and reference, especially for home care and primary care providers. A comprehensive bibliography at the end of the chapter provides additional sources of authoritative information.

138. Wetle T. (1991). Successful aging: New hope for optimizing mental and physical well-being. _J Geront Psychiatry_, _24_(1):3-12.

The author addresses four myths regarding aging and demonstrates how these myths, when accepted, promote negative and destructive feelings about the elderly. The premise used is that much of what was once thought to be inevitable and irreversible is, today, preventable or treatable. The article provides helpful insights regarding attitudes toward older persons.

139. Witte M. (1989). Pain control. _J Geront Nurs_, _15_(3):32-37.

Older persons' perception of pain are likely to vary, depending on overall health status and presence of multiple health problems. Physiological changes that occur along with aging play an important role, particularly with regard to reaction to narcotics and analgesics. Recommended for care providers and pharmacists.

140. Wright G. (1991). Geropharmacology: An individualized approach. _J Amer Acad Nurs Practitioners_, _3_(2):85-89.

Drug therapy in the elderly presents many problems requiring approaches tailored to the individual's status and needs. Factors to be considered include age, physiological and psychological status, and specific responses to drugs based on observation and foundational knowledge about normal physiologic changes that occur in aging, and about the pharmacokinetic and pharmacodynamic mechanisms of iatrogenic drug reactions. Social and ethical issues related to drugs also need to be kept in mind.

141. Yazdanfar D. J. (1990). Assessing the mental status of the cognitively impaired elderly. _J Geront Nurs_, _16_(9):32-36.

Loneliness and isolation among homebound elderly often

result in confusion and other evidences of changing mental status. Care providers need to make periodic assessment of cognitive abilities to enable individuals to function optimally. Recommended for practitioners and caregivers who work closely with elderly clients in any setting.

B. Housing:

142. Blank T. O. (1988). Older Persons and Their Housing Today and Tomorrow. Springfield, IL: Charles C. Thomas Publishers.

Although this book covers all aspects of housing, including types, ownership, insurance, equity, and design, it also discusses home care, family caregivers, and other areas relating to health care in the home, making it a valuable addition to the literature about home health care of the elderly. Recommended for policy planners, housing planners, families, and practitioners.

143. Muller C. (1989). Shared housing for the elderly. In Health Care of the Elderly: An Information Sourcebook. M. D. Petersen, D. L. White (eds.). Newbury Park, CA: Sage Publications, 329-381.

Research done on shared housing reveals that financial savings is the one factor shown to be a measurable positive outcome. Other effects may result, but current research methods have not been able to discriminate these and other variables, such as activities of daily living (ADL) abilities, reduced use of health care services, and changed health status. Comprehensive information and ideas for future research in this area.

144. Rabin D. L., Davis A. R. (1989). New community options for elderly patients. In Clinical Aspects of Aging, 3rd Ed. W. Reichel (ed.) Baltimore: Williams & Wilkins, 518-528.

Most Americans at any age prefer to be independent and autonomous, able to care for themselves. The content in this chapter defines and describes various living arrangements that promote independence in the elderly. Costs of alternative housing and Medicare and Medicaid support are addressed, indicating that less than 2% of Medicaid expenditures are for home health care. Excellent overview of housing situations for older persons who can remain independent.

145. Redfoot D. L. (1991). Coordinating housing and services for the elderly. Caring, 10(5):44-51.

Major new housing legislation, the National Affordable Housing Act, greatly increases the possibilities for the frail elderly to maintain their independence by remaining at home. The emphasis on connecting services and housing is particularly significant. Some of the kinds of assistance that this legislation will make possible are home repairs, service-enriched vouchers, and congregate services.

146. Regnier V., Pynoos J. (1987). Housing the Aged: Design Directives and Policy Considerations. New York: Elsevier Science Publishing Company, Inc.

The authors discuss housing policy issues, planned housing for the well elderly, supportive housing for the moderately impaired, and environments for the frail elderly. Although the emphasis is housing, content includes a variety of information, all focusing on home care. Among these topics are ways that people can and do change their behaviors to cope with increasing disability, and disability assessment tools. Recommended for policy planners, architects who are required to design elderly housing, families, and practitioners.

147. Rollinson P. A. (1991). Elderly single room occupancy (SRO) hotel tenants: still alone. Soc Work, 36(4):303-308.

A disproportionate number of urban poor elderly people live in what has been characterized as the nation's least desirable housing stock--single room occupancy (SRO) hotels. A study was conducted in hotels of a

Chicago neighborhood, with data collected on the everyday experiences of 53 elderly tenants. The findings showed that this type of housing does not foster independence. Many subjects indicated that they felt trapped in a situation that exacerbated their isolation. Many were in desperate need of social services.

148. Shore H. (1989). Housing for the elderly. In Clinical Aspects of Aging, 3rd ed. W. Reichel (ed.) Baltimore: Williams and Wilkins, 510-517.

The emphasis is housing for the elderly, since the environment should promote the physical and mental well-being by providing opportunities for socialization and health maintenance, while permitting privacy and the continuation of one's accustomed lifestyle. Content includes decisions about relocation and the possible effects of moving, kinds of available and desired housing, and financial aspects of ownership, rental, and other forms of possession.

149. Struyk R. J., Katsura H. M. (1988). Aging at Home: How the Elderly Adjust Their Housing Without Moving. Binghamton, NY: Haworth Press.

Adjustments that older persons must make in order to remain at home are presented in this unique book: changing the use of rooms, modifying structures to accommodate the impaired or frail elderly, and taking in roomers. Recommended for caregivers and families with older members.

150. Tell E. J., Cohen M. A. (1990). Continuing-care retirement communities. Generations:55-59, spring.

Lessons in managing costs of long-term care in continuing care retirement communities is discussed. Highlighted is the need to provide some kind of long-term care cost protection in these retirement communities in order to remain competitive with the consumer. Information discussed is relevant for home health care providers since they are often asked about living arrangements by their clients and families.

C. Adult Day Care:

151. Graham R. W. (1989). Adult day care: How families of the dementia patient respond. J Geront Nurs, 15(3): 27-31.

Caring for family members with dementia in the home is a physical, emotional, and financial strain for most caregivers. Responses to adult day care were varied and complex, indicating mixed reactions. The need for additional research about this kind of care is evident.

152. Tate L. A., Brennan C. M. (1988). Adult Day Care. Binghamton, NY: Haworth Press.

Information provided includes the history, definition, and concept of day care, models of care, scope of activities, state and national policies, and samples of forms and reports needed for operating/assessing these facilities. Excellent resource for administrators of adult day care centers and interested others.

D. Nutrition:

153. All New Cookbook for Diabetics and Their Families. Binghamton, NY: Haworth Press.

This is a sequel to Cookbook for Diabetics and Their Families, published several years ago. This new edition has virtually all new recipes, with consideration given to preparation and calories, cholesterol, and cost of ingredients. Many of the recipes are simple as well as appealing to diminished taste in the elderly. Anyone who must pay strict attention to dietary intake will find this cookbook well worth owning.

154. Easton P. S., Harker C. S. et al (1991). Nutrition Care of People With Diabetes Mellitus. Binghamton, NY: Haworth Press.

A nutrition reference book for health professionals that features practical advice based on sound and scientific data about care of diabetes. Suggestions about controlling food intake and how to live with this chronic disease should prove valuable to practitioners and clients alike.

155. Gallagher-Allred C. (1991). Nutrition and the elderly. Caring, 10(5):68-72.

A variety of factors--psychological, sociological, and economic--relate to older persons suffering the consequences of malnutrition. Some of the causes of decreased or inappropriate balance of nutritional food include decrease in appetite, decreased sense perceptions of taste and smell, difficulties in chewing and swallowing, anorexia caused by depression and loneliness, and physical problems that interfere with the body's ability to digest or absorb food. Screening for nutrition problems is therefore particularly necessary in elderly patients being cared for at home.

156. Hall M. (1986). Study of Registered Dietitians' Services in Home Care. Washington, DC: Policy Information Center, ID# 2185.

Congress ordered a study of the circumstances and conditions under which Title 18 of the Social Security Act should cover dietitians' services as a home health care benefit. This report discusses the need for these services and explores alternative methods for coverage and reimbursement. Content also includes estimates of utilization rates and financial costs of the services. Excellent background information regarding meeting elderly clients' nutritional needs.

157. Hogstel M. O., Robinson N. D. (1989). Feeding the frail elderly. J Geront Nurs, 15(3):16-20.

Careful observation, appropriate foods, and the right utensils are important in assisting frail older persons to take in sufficient nourishment safely. Problems with swallowing, loss of teeth, choking, and aspirating need to be monitored. Excellent resource for caregivers of the old-old.

158. Tong A. (1991). Eating habits of elderly Vietnamese in the United States. J Nutr for Elderly, 10(2):35-48.

About 39,500 Vietnamese refugees and immigrants came to the US in 1975. Many of this group are now getting older. In a sample of 62 elderly Vietnamese, the investigators used a 24-hour recall to examine food habits and incidence of common diseases. This helpful article makes practitioner and nutritionists aware of the special needs of Asian and other populations new to the United States.

159. Zumwalt S., Schmidt R. M. (1989). In AIDS and aging: The role of nutrition. Generations:77-79, fall.

The importance of nutrition in both the elderly and those affected by the human immunodeficiency virus (HIV/AIDS) has not been sufficiently emphasized in either group. Malnutrition is explored because of maldigestion and malabsorption problems that are common in both populations. Major goals for good nutritional management are outlined. Recommended for caregivers and care providers.

E. Minority Populations:

160. Applewhite S. R. (1988). Hispanic Elderly in Transition: Theory, Research, Policy and Practice. Westport, CT: Greenwood Press.

This book addresses the health, economic, social, and cultural issues influencing the quality of life among older Hispanics in the U.S. There are five parts, each of which addresses particular areas: 1) cultural, historical, and sociodemographic aspects of the Hispanic population, 2) health status and health service utilization, 3) politics and public policy, political empowerment, and income maintenance for elderly Hispanic people, 4) family, community, and natural support systems, and 5) research on elderly Hispanic groups. Recommended for care providers, researchers, and others whose focus is the elderly Hispanic population.

161. Harel Z., McKinney E. A., Williams M. (eds.) (1990). Black Aged: Understanding Diversity and Service Needs. Newbury Park, CA: Sage Publications.

This volume is published in cooperation with the National Council on Aging, Inc. It offers comparisons of various ethnic communities on levels of health, income, and quality of housing for their elders. Conceptual perspectives are provided on the uniqueness of black aged as a group and analytical approaches about understanding diversity are discussed.

162. Health care needs of the minority elderly. Caring, 10(5):58-61.

This article was excerpted from Empowerment of Minority Elderly: Conference and Roundtable Discussions, published by the American Association of Retired Persons (AARP), Washington, DC, 1990. The AARP has compiled data that provides the information contained in a document, "A Portrait of Older Minorities." The research shows that, largely because of cultural differences, minority elderly are not as likely to participate in health services as are white elderly. The same tendency is prevalent among American Indians. Both groups tend to defer seeking care except in serious acute illnesses or for debilitating long-term illnesses. Health professionals need to be aware of cultural differences which affect use of health care services.

163. Henderson G. (1989). A Practitioner's Guide to Understanding Indigenous and Foreign Cultures. Springfield, IL: Charles C. Thomas Publishers.

Although the practitioner focus in this book is the psychotherapist, the same principles apply to all those who interact with people from many cultures. The author provides a strong rationale for the need to understand other cultures, while stating that "no person is an exact representation of his or her culture at any given time." While the content includes a large amount of helpful information, there is no overall theoretical framework which would help to organize and link the array of facts.

164. Lewin-Epstein N. (1991). Determinants of regular source of health care in black, Mexican, Puerto Rican, and non-Hispanic white populations. Medical Care, 29(6):543-557.

Access to care for underserved minorities, while it has improved in the past twenty years, is still a matter of serious concern, particularly for poor and ethnic minorities. Use of hospital emergency room and outpatient departments by these groups has been growing, which results in further increasing the cost of health care overall. This study examined specific determinants derived from data sets of patients living in poverty areas of Chicago. While there was variance among the groups, with Mexicans least likely to have a regular source of care, all received minimal care. The problems are confounded for elderly minorities, resulting in more social isolation.

165. Sotomayor M., Curiel H. (1988). Hispanic Elderly: A Cultural Signature. Edinburg, TX: Pan American University Press.

This is a comprehensive analysis of the Hispanic culture to enable the reader to more fully understand and appreciate the Spanish heritage, the past and current cultural milieux, and the Hispanic values and beliefs. Valuable resource for all those who interact with Hispanic people in any setting.

166. Taukashira Y. (1988). Reaching out to families of the Asian elderly. Aging, no. 358:11-13.

Asian refugees and immigrants, particularly those who are older, experience culture shock, disorientation, isolation, and loneliness. Social service agencies can enhance the quality of their lives in many ways: providing information, disseminating materials in many languages, establishing community forums, and using the ethnic churches to reach those who may be homebound and chronically ill. The Asian Human Care Centers, 5211 W. Olympic Boulevard, Los Angeles, CA, 90036, will send fact sheets and brochures that describe their services and networks.

F. Case Management:

167. Austin C. D., O'Connor K. (1989). Case management: Components and program contexts. In: M.D. Petersen, D.L. White (eds.). Health Care of the Elderly: Information Sourcebook. Newbury Park, CA: Sage Publications, 167-205.

The multiple needs of frail elders for comprehensive in-home services and the complexity of the health care system support the need for case managers who coordinate the services of several providers, advocate for client needs and rights, and serve as gatekeepers to control costs of services.

168. Challis D., Darton R., Johnson L., Stone M., Traske K. (1991). An evaluation of an alternative to long-stay hospital care for frail elderly patients: I. The model of care. Age and Ageing, 20:236-244.

Recent United Kingdom government policy has advocated the development of case management to provide more coordinated care at home for vulnerable people. This paper describes a service model where case managers, with devolved budgets, employed by the social services department, were placed with a multidisciplinary team to provide an alternative for patients requiring long-stay hospital care. The role of the case manager in the team is described, and the tasks undertaken by home care assistants are delineated. Home care assistants undertook a wider range of activities than either home helps or nurses, covering both personal and domestic care tasks.

169. Challis D., Darton R., Johnson L., Stone M., Traske K. (1991). An evaluation of an alternative to

long-stay hospital care for frail elderly patients: II. Costs and effectiveness. Age and Ageing, 20:245-254.

This paper continues the description of an alternative model of care for frail elderly, other than long-stay hospitalization. The main findings of the evaluation, using elderly people who received the service as the experimental group, and a group of similar patients who did not receive the case management services as the control group. Findings showed that the experimental group had a higher quality of life, and there was no evidence of greater stress on their caregivers. The community-based service, although it involved extra costs to the social services department, had lower costs for the total health service and society as a whole than long-stay hospital care. It is concluded that the model of care can effectively integrate the new approach of case management into an existing geriatric multidisciplinary team.

170. Kane R. A., Penrod J. D., Davidson G., Moscovice I. (1991). What cost case management in long-term care? Soc Serv Rev, 65(2):281-303.

Data from a sample of 48 case management programs were reviewed, and showed variation in program characteristics and costs. Case management varied in practice and in ways that affect both the cost of case management itself and the costs of services being managed. However, virtually no relationship was found between costs and client characteristics, client outcomes, or case management inputs. Implications for research and policy in case management in long-term care are discussed.

171. Korr W. S., Cloninger L. (1991). Assessing models of case management: an empirical approach. J Soc Serv Res, 14(1/2):129-146.

No research has been done on whether different models of case management are being implemented. This study focused on case management services provided to chronically mentally ill elderly, and assessed whether the case management followed any or all of the models postulated by Ross (1980) - Minimal, Coordination, or Comprehensive. Data analysis showed that case management services were given according to all three models. Implications for case management practice and for research are presented.

172. Oleson M., King T. W. (1990). Back to the beginning: Nursing case management of the older client with alaryngeal speech needs. J Geront Nurs, 16(12):27-29.

Loss of speech because of laryngectomy is a severe trauma in many older persons' lives. A case manager can muster and coordinate support from various sources to ensure that alaryngeal speech becomes effectively established through special aids and training. A speech-language pathologist/therapist is vital to this goal.

173. Putney K. A., Hauner J., Hall T., Kobb R. (1990). Case management in long-term care: New directions for professional nursing. J Geront Nurse, 16(12):30-33.

Although the nursing home is the setting, the principles of case management with older persons can be effectively applied in the home with equally positive outcomes: quality of care that is cost-effective, and satisfaction and independence for patients.

174. Wood L. (1991). Geriatric case management: The time is now. J Geront Nurs, 17(4):3.

The concern in this editorial is meeting the health and social needs of the ever-increasing population of frail elderly in communities. The author proposes that gerontological nurses assume the role of case managers to ensure efficient and cost-effective comprehensive delivery of care to meet physical, psychological, and social needs directly and by means of appropriate consultation with and referral to other health care team members.

G. Health Care Providers:

175. Brannon D., Smyer M. A. (1990). Who will provide long-term care in the future? Generations:64-67, spring.

A thorough discussion of personnel projections to meet the growing long-term care needs of the future, both in nursing homes and in home health agencies, is provided. Intensified competition for all levels and types of health care workers is projected. Strategies for consideration in planning for these needs are discussed and have potentially critical implications for the future of long-term care financing, administration, and quality of care for the elderly.

176. Genevay B., Katz R. S. (1990). Counter-transference and Older Clients. Newbury Park, CA: Sage Publications.

Useful suggestions are provided for dealing constructively with our emotional reactions as health professionals when working with older adults. Numerous case studies are presented about how our own desires and capacity to be therapeutic agents to our elderly clients can affect quality of care. Important topics included are terminal illness and death, suicidal elders, disability, and AIDS. Excellent resource for orienting new staff in particular to the rigors of caring for vulnerable populations.

4

Caregivers

177. Alley J. M. (1988). Family Caregiving: Family Strains, Coping Response Patterns, and Caregiving Burden. Doctoral dissertation. Virginia Polytechnic Institute and State University.

This study addressed gaps in the literature on caregiver burden involving lack of information about the multiple strains on caregiving families, their coping patterns, and positive as well as negative aspects of caregiving. The primary objective was to examine the relationship among caregiving strains, patterns of coping responses employed, and the resulting subjective and objective caregiver burden. Implications for practice include the importance of health workers considering multiple sources of strain in the family.

178. Barusch A. S. (1991). Elder Care: Family Training and Support. Newbury Park, CA: Sage Publications.

The first half of this book explores a full range of topics on support programs for family caregivers. The second half focuses on the Wellsprings Training Program at the University of Utah's Caregiver Support Project providing indepth coverage of common concerns such as medication management, power of attorney, home safety, self-care, and other relevant areas.

179. Barusch A. S., Spaid W. M. (1991). Reducing caregiver burden through short-term training: Evaluation

findings from a caregiver support project. J Geront Soc Work, 17(1/2):7-33.

A Caregiver Support Project was established to develop and evaluate training interventions for older spouse caregivers. A total of 113 caregivers participated in six weekly sessions designed to enhance their coping skills and reduce their sense of burden. Results indicate that the intervention improved coping responses and slightly reduced caregiver burden. Family participation in training enhanced the impact of the training.

180. Berger R., Anderson S. (1984). The in-home worker: serving the frail elderly. Social Work, 29(5):456-461.

This article focuses on the interpersonal problems that in-home providers working with frail elderly must often cope with. Based on a systematic assessment of the problems, a typology of situations is presented accompanied by guidelines for the training, assessment, and supervision of workers and their clients in the home setting. A unique resource for educators of home care providers and caregivers.

181. Biegel D. E., Blum A. (1990). Aging and Caregiving: Theory, Research, and Policy. Newbury Park, CA: Sage Focus Editions, Volume 110.

Health care professionals and educators will find this book useful in their work with older adults and their caregivers. The volume focuses on research findings, on theories of caregiving, and on public policy concerns from an international perspective. Outstanding resource for those working in this field.

182. Briggs L., Carroccio J. (1991). Seniors caring for seniors: Expanding eldercare services. Caring, 10(5):74-76.

The Visiting Nurse Associations of America (VNAAs) are spearheading a national demonstration project aimed at creating collaborative partnerships between nonprofit, community-based VNAs and the Senior Companion Program to expand the scope of person-to-person volunteer programs and long-term care services. This article describes the project design and purposes. Excellent presentation of innovative strategies to promote collaboration among groups to enhance care for the elderly.

183. Brody E. M. (1990). Women in the Middle: Their Parent-Care Years. New York: Springer Publishing Company.

The author has devoted a significant portion of her career to investigating the effect of parent care on the lives of women. These women are frequently caught in the middle because of multiple roles and responsibilties that compete for time and energy, dichotomous values regarding caring for parents and the need for a career, and the almost inevitable tensions between the elderly parents and other family members. Many aspects of this increasingly important problem are addressed in this comprehensive book.

184. Brown L. J., Potter J. F., Foster B. G. (1990). Caregiver burden should be evaluated during geriatric assessment. J Amer Geriatr Soc, 30(4):465-60.

This article stresses the need for the care provider to do a comprehensive assessment of the home situation at the time the initial history and physical examination are done, to determine the potential impact of the older person's illness or disability on the family members who are or will be caregivers, and to assess total resources available to the patient. A detailed outline regarding assessment is included.

185. Buchsbaum S. (1991). Sending "care" packages to the workplace. Business & Health, 9(5):56-69.

About 5500 companies have policies that assist employees who need day care for preschool children. Many of these companies, such as Stride-Rite in Cambridge, Massachusetts, are expanding day care facilities for children to include eldercare programs for those workers who have responsibility for older parents. Some companies, rather than provide on-site centers for dependent children and relatives, grant paid time off to allow employees to give care. Other modes of employer cooperation in meeting worker's needs include flex-time, family leave policies, and flex-place, which allows employees to work at home. Studies of at-home workers show that they are at least as productive as those in the work setting.

186. Bush M. (1987). Characteristics and Needs of Black Caregivers and Their Elderly Clients in Personal Care Homes. Washington, DC: Policy Information Center, ID# 3218.

Research findings are included in this final report of a study conducted by the American Red Cross and the Congress of National Black Churches on the needs and characteristics of caregivers and their black elderly clients in community-based personal care homes. Ways are identified to strengthen caregivers' support of the black elderly in these arrangements through local and national Red Cross centers, government agencies, volunteer organizations, and local churches.

187. Caserta M. et al (1987). Caregivers to dementia patients: The utilization of community services. Gerontologist, 27(2):209-214.

This article centers on the types of services most used by caregivers in providing care to persons with dementia, and the factors that influence use of particular services. Respite services were seen as most needed and were most utilized. Perceived caregiver burden, level of involvement with the care of the demented person, and availability of resources all affected caregiver choices of appropriate services. Valuable resource for administrators of home care agencies, trainers of caregivers, and providers of home care.

188. Cicirelli V. G. (1991). Family Caregiving: Autonomous and Paternalistic Decision Making. Newbury Park, CA: Sage Publications. Sage Library of Social Research, Volume 186.

Answers are provided to questions posed by researchers, practitioners, and professionals regarding how authoritarian family traditions and negative attitudes toward the elderly affect the frequency of paternalistic decision making and the quality of family caregiving. Unique to this book is its emphasis on respect for autonomy in family caregiving and decision making.

189. Colman V. et al (1987). Till Death Do Us Part: Caregiving Wives of Severely Disabled Husbands. ERIC, # ED320058.

This paper describes the problems encountered by wives in a caregiving role for severely incapacitated husbands. It identifies problems in the present health care delivery system that contribute to this situation. These include the limitations of Medicare, Medicaid, and other sources of assistance such as Social Security, private insurance coverage, and private nursing agencies. The paper includes strategies to assist in coping with these difficulties.

190. Corbin J. M., Strauss A. (1988). Unending Care and Work: Managing Chronic Illness at Home. San Francisco, CA: Jossey-Bass Publishers.

Understanding the course and impact of chronic illness, managing chronic illness, assisting in the recovery and maintenance phases, coping with disequilibrium and downward stages of illness, and other similar topics are detailed in this informative book, which should prove particularly helpful for caregivers and health care workers in the home setting.

191. Cranston A. (1990). Work and family: Public policy issues for the 1990s. Families in Society: J of Contemp Human Services 71:360-365.

This California senator addresses the needs of families in today's society in which, primarily because of economic necessity, both partners must work. The demands of the work place added stress in those families where members must also care for older parents. Many aspects of family needs and problems are discussed in this article.

192. Creedon M. A. (1988). The corporate response to the working caregivers. Aging, no. 358:16-19, 45.

Research studies on employers and eldercare showed that a large number of employees--20-30%--have responsibility for caring for one or both elderly parents. A 1987 report by the National Association of Area Agencies on Aging (NAAAA) indicated the average time that caregivers provided care was about 15.9 hours per week. Types of care included transportation, personal care, making appointments, providing meals, home maintenance, completing various forms, searching for new residence, and financial assistance. Many caregivers are caught between the need to work and the demands of caregiving. Some employers respond by sponsoring support groups, caregiver forums, information, and counseling.

193. Denton K., Love L. T., Slate R. (1990). Eldercare in the '90s: Employee responsibility, employer challenge. Families in Society: The J of Contemp Human Services, 71(6):349-359.

Americans are living longer, but the family members who traditionally care for our elderly--women--now constitute well over half of all new employees. To identify trends in supports offered by employers to workers who are caring for elderly relatives, representatives of 20 employers were interviewed. The responses showed that while employers appreciate the burdens of workers with eldercare responsibility, they have not systematically examined their employees' problems or developed policies to address those needs. Policy implications of these findings are discussed.

194. Doherty E. S., Power P. W. (1990). Identifying the needs of coronary patient wife-caregivers: Implications for social workers. Health and Social Work, 15(4):291-299.

Ninety-three women responded to a mail questionnaire

regarding needs directly or indirectly created by their husbands' major medical crises involving coronary heart disease. Three areas of strong needs were identified: education, prevention, and support services. These needs have implications for health care professionals' interventions with wife-caregivers in assessing, planning, and interpersonal relationships. To ensure optimal outcomes, the needs of the caregiver as well as the patient must be met.

195. Farran C. J., Keane-Hagerty E. (1991). An interactive model for finding meaning through caregiving. In: Anthology on Caring, P. L. Chinn (ed.). New York: National League for Nursing, Publ. # 15-2392, 225-237.

In recent years, increased research has been conducted with family caregivers of the elderly. To date, no theoretical frameworks exclusively devoted to family caregiving have emerged. The literature on caregiving seems to emphasize negative aspects of the role. This chapter focuses on a model that provides direction toward more positive perspectives and outcomes for the caregiver. The model is based on Frankl's work: 1) persons create meaning by making choices, 2) values provide the basis for meaning, 3) each person has the responsibility for right action and conduct, and 4) there are two levels of meaning: provisional and ultimate. Unique resource for home care providers.

196. Hamilton L. A., Jones H. C. (1986). The "Unidentified Patient" in Home Health Care. ERIC, # ED294075.

This paper was presented at the annual meeting of the National Association of Social Workers and describes the role and problems of women who provide home care for elderly spouses, parents, and other family members. Many of these women have chronic conditions themselves and the existing health care system does little to provide status or care for these "unidentified patients."

197. Heagerty B., Dunn L., Watson M. A. (1988). Helping caregivers care. Aging, no. 358:7-10.

When illness of an aged person occurs, family members often find themselves thrust into roles they are not prepared to assume. The profound physical, psychological, social, and financial changes brought about by chronic illness or impairment can adversely affect the entire family. This article focuses on the assistance provided by the Education and Family Support Services (E&FSS) of the Good Samaritan Hospital and Medical Center in Portland, Oregon. Such help can significantly enhance the coping abilities of caregivers.

198. Heery K. (1991). Eldercare: The challenge of the '90s. Caring, 10(5):62-64.

The demands of caring for an aging parent are often great, especially when caregivers work and are responsible for other family members. Many elderly have complex needs and multiple health problems that often include disability. Health care professionals are in a key position to evaluate the feasibility of eldercare in a given situation, to recommend treatment alternatives, and to counsel caregivers who may be overwhelmed.

199. Jacob S. R. (1991). Support for family caregivers in the community. Fam Community Health, 14(1):16-21.

Family caregivers are playing an increasingly prominent role in providing care to older relatives - spouses or parents. These caregivers face a variety of stresses. Health care professionals must understand the caregiver's burden to intervene effectively and promote healthy adaptation to stress. Partnerships between caregivers and care providers should be nurtured to facilitate essential support and education for the family, caregivers, and patients.

200. Kaye L. W. (1985). Home care for the aged: A fragile partnership. Social Work, 30(4):312-317.

This article describes the efforts of formal and informal caregivers who provide services for the homebound elderly. The conclusion is that informal support is preferred for most home care services. Formal support was preferred for housekeeping, specialized chores, and repetitive tasks. Excellent resource for health care professionals, home care agency administrators, and caregivers.

201. Kaye L. W., Applegate J. S. (1991). Components of a gender-sensitive curriculum model for elder caregiving: Lessons from research. Gerontology and Geriatrics Education, 11(3):39-56.

Students in the helping professions need to learn gender-sensitive practice approaches to service delivery in order to respond to the changing needs of family members providing care to frail elderly parents and relatives. This article presents a summary of a national study of male caregivers. Findings from research about the complexity of family caregiving patterns that span the generations provide the foundation for developing classroom content and practicum experiences. Recommended for curriculum planners and faculty who teach this content.

202. Klein S. M. (1986). In-Home Respite Care for Older Adults: A Guide for Program Planners, Administrators, and Clinicians. Springfield, IL: Charles C. Thomas Publisher.

This comprehensive manual is divided into four areas: administering a respite program; tracking and reporting information about clients, families, providers; training volunteers; forms and data collection. The manual contains handouts, teaching guidelines, examples of forms for recordkeeping, and other useful materials.

203. Lamy P. P., Gondek K. et al (1991). The family caregiver. Elder Care News, 7(3). Baltimore: University of Maryland School of Pharmacy.

This is a report from the Maryland Caregivers Programs that provides a comprehensive review of the multidimensional aspects of providing care for the elderly and the primary role of the family caregiver. Of particular note is the fact that the family caregiver makes important decisions on behalf of the elderly more than half the time, rather than the patient or the health care provider, as is often thought. An interesting and informative article reflecting the need of the caregiver to be informed and able to extend care that is safe and comprehensive.

204. Lynch-Sauer J. (1990). When a family member has Alzheimer's disease: A phenomenological description of caregiving. J Geront Nurs, 16(9):8-11.

The caregiving relationship is dynamic. Factors related to the optimal well-being of both receiver and giver of care include the situational context, the degree of interaction possible between patient and caregiver, and the quality of the relationship. Specific and useful resource for caregivers and families.

205. Montgomery R. (1989). Respite services for family caregivers. In Health Care of the Elderly: An Information Sourcebook. Eds.: M. D. Petersen, D. L. White. Newbury Park, CA: Sage Publications, Inc., 382-410.

This chapter presents a systematic collection of integrated information about models of respite services, the benefits of these models for family caregivers, and the impact of respite services on caregiving behaviors. Findings have implications for administrators and providers of care in nursing homes and home care agencies, and for researchers.

206. National Institutes of Health Consensus Development Conference (1990). The Treatment of Sleep Disorders of Older People. Bethesda, MD: Office of Medical Applications of Research, volume 8, no. 3.

Clinical specialists in pulmonary, psychiatry, psychology, geriatrics, and internal medicine were brought together to address the causes, diagnosis, assessment, and specific treatments of sleep disorders in older people. The findings presented during the conference are reported in this publication.

207. Norris J. (ed.) (1988). Daughters of the Elderly: Building Partnerships in Caregiving. Bloomington, IL: Indiana University Press.

Useful information on how to care for elderly parents, options to be considered, and a feeling for the caregiver/parent relationship are provided in this volume. Various circumstances are described in personal narrative form by the primary caregivers. Health professionals should find this book useful in understanding these relationships and in providing support to the elderly and to their caregivers in an effective and sensitive manner.

208. Opie N. D., Miller E. T. (1989). Attribution for successful relationships between severely disabled adults and personal care attendants. Rehabilit Nurs, 14(4):196-99.

This study explored disabled adults and their personal care attendants regarding their definitions of the relationship and causal explanations for the relationship outcome (either success or failure). Attribution theory was used to shape the study design. The most frequently cited explanations for a successful outcome were mutual effort, skill, and commitment of the personal care attendant and disabled adult. The majority of subjects defined their relationship as productive and friendly.

209. Osterkamp L. (1988). Family caregiver: America's primary long-term care resource. Aging, no. 358:2-6.

To help caregivers effectively, a profile is needed of who they are, how they manage, what problems they face, and what types of assistance they need. Based on survey results, the author found that there are about 2.2 million unpaid caregivers, with the average caregiver a woman, age 55-60. One-third of the respondents were over 65. The frail person's spouse is the most likely to become the caregiver. Wives of severely impaired men provide the most informal care. The majority said that their needs included education and training, emotional support, relief from financial strain, and to know that others care about them and what they are doing.

210. Primomo J., Yates B. C., Woods N. F. (1990). Social support for women during chronic illness: The relationship among sources and types to adjustment. Res Nurs & Health, 13(3):153-161.

Findings show that women perceive more support from partners than from other family members and friends. Types of support included affect, affirmation, and reciprocity; these related to less depression, higher marital quality, and better family functioning.

211. Printz-Feddersen V. (1990). Group process effect on caregiver burden. J Neurosci Nurs, 22(3):164-68.

This ex-post facto study examines the burden experience of people caring for a stroke survivor. One hypothesis was that there would be less caregiver burden in those caregivers who participated in a stroke club (experimental) than those who did not (control). Measurement was done by using the CADET to evaluate functional status of the stroke survivor, the Physical Caregiving Responsibility Inventory for the degree of difficulty performing caregiving experiences, and the Geriatric Depression Scale for degree of caregiver depression. Factors having the most influence to decrease the effect of caregiving burden were: 1) advanced educational background, 2) high income, and 3) patient's moderate physical disabilities.

212. Reifler B. V., Henry R. S., Sherrill K. (1990). National dementia care and respite services program. Generations:70-71, spring.

A description of the Robert Wood Johnson Foundation's National Dementia Care and Respite Services Program is provided in this article. The goals of the program include 1) to expand the availability of day programs for people with dementia, and other community and in-home respite services; 2) to demonstrate that these day centers can provide and coordinate needed services, and 3) to determine whether these services can be provided on a financially viable basis. A history of the development of day care centers is also provided.

213. Riebschleger J. L. (1991). Families of chronically mentally ill people: Siblings speak to social workers. Health & Social Work, 16(2):94-103.

Twenty siblings of chronically mentally ill people discussed their emotional responses to the mental illness of their brother or sister. These responses were categorized into phases of the grieving process (denial, anger, bargaining, depression, relief/respite, and acceptance. The siblings recommended including them in client treatment. Needs identified were support, education of family members, clear communication between social worker and family, a focus on family strengths, and effective interventions in client treatment and care.

214. St. George J., Dicicco-Bloom B. (1985). Using dramatization to train caregivers for the elderly. Nursing Outlook, 33(6):302-304.

Role-playing is discussed as a strategy for home health aides, who can use this strategy to focus on common problems found in the setting, and on how to work with elderly persons. Unusual and useful resource for administrators of home care agencies and providers of care in the home.

215. Schirm V. (1990). Shared caregiving responsibilities for chronically ill elders. Holistic Nurs Pract, 5(1):54-61.

The author examines the concept of shared caregiving in which the goal is to develop a balanced and coordinated relationship among the elderly care recipients, family caregivers, and practitioners. The result is sharing of functions between informal and formal caregiving systems. Experiences of home care providers show that interventions by professionals that complement the tasks already being done by family caregivers enhance outcomes for elderly care recipients.

216. Schneider E. L. (ed.) (1989). Handbook of the Biology of Aging, 3rd Edition. San Diego, CA: Academic Press.

This new edition provides a comprehensive overview of some of the most important topics in biomedical gerontology. It updates previous editions and covers new advances in geriatric medicine, neurobiology of aging, and Alzheimer's disease research.

217. Steinmetz S. K. (1988). Family and Support Systems Across the Life Span. New York: Plenum Press.

This is a collection of articles focusing on the role that families and formal systems play in providing social support for individuals at various points across the lifespan continuum. One author contends that the family continues to play the most important role in providing support, whether the family is a single unit or separate members. This is a helpful reference for families, clients, and providers of care to the elderly in home and community settings.

218. Vinick B. H., Ekerdt D. J. (1991). Retirement: What happens to husband-wife relationships? J Geriatr Psychiatry, 24(1):13-40.

Research conducted with 92 couples indicates that retirement does not typically result in major changes in the lives of married couples. While some stress may occur initially, solutions are sought by both spouses and the stress dissipates quickly. Virtually no study of nonclinical populations demonstrates a strong negative impact of retirement on the quality of the marriage.

219. Walker A. J., Pratt C. C., Martell L. K., Martin S. S. K. (1991). Perceptions of aid and actual aid in intergenerational caregiving. Fam Relations, 40(3):318-323.

In this study, 174 pairs of elderly mothers and their caregiving daughters were compared as to the perceptions of each with respect to aid given to the mothers, with reports of actual caregiving activities performed. Just over half of the women overestimated the amount of aid given, while most of the remainder perceived it accurately. Highly educated and younger mothers had more accurate perceptions than poorly educated and older mothers. Daughters who perceived their mothers to be in better health and who lived separately had more accurate perceptions than daughters who saw their mothers' health as poor and who resided with them. The discussion emphasizes the high level of accurate perceptions among both mothers and daughters.

220. Wayne State University (1987). Effects of Alternative Family Support Strategies. Washington, DC: Policy Information Center, PIC ID# 3685.

The cost of custodial care and the increase in the number of impaired older persons have stimulated interest in services supporting families in their role as caregivers. A total of 541 units participated in this experimentally designed study that investigated the impact of family support programs which included the provisions of training and respite services. The final report provides information regarding significantly different outcomes from the varied combinations of support services offered.

221. Wernig J. K., Sorrentino S. A. (1989). The Homemaker-Home Health Aide. St. Louis: Mosby.

Contents include basic essential information on such topics as home care, communications, needs of clients, how the body functions, safety and controlling infection in the home, and home maintenance. This comprehensive text is intended for individuals with little educational or experiential background in home care.

222. The Womanly World of Long-Term Care: The Plight of the Long-Term Care Worker, (1989). Washington, DC: Older Women's League. ERIC # ED 318902.

This paper describes the problems of workers who are

paid to provide custodial care to imcreasing numbers of elderly persons in homes as well as nursing homes. The home health aide needs increased training for competency, and salaries are low. This workforce is primarily female. The common use of the medical model that categorizes care as "skilled" or "custodial" places these workers in the latter category, thus perpetuating their low status in a field that requires continuing increases in both quality and quantity of care.

5

Administration

223. Ammentorp W., Gossett K. D., Poe N. E. (1991). Quality Assurance for Long-Term Care Providers. Newbury Park, CA: Sage Publications.

A clear explanation of the OBRA regulations of 1987 is provided in this book. Health care professionals, who provide consultation and referral services to elderly clients, their caregivers, and other health care professionals will find the plan presented to be a useful reference for complying with evolving regulations in the long-term care arena.

224. Arikian V. L. (1991). Total quality management: applications to nursing service. J Nurs Admin, 21(6):46-50.

Total quality management (TQM) can offer practical solutions to the new economic mode of "best for less" when specifically adapted to the needs of the nursing profession and individual nursing administration areas. The author describes the TQM philosophy and principles, presents strategies that may be used by nurse executives to integrate TQM into their management systems, and discusses specific guidelines for successful implementation of TQM.

225. Beland F. (1986). The clientele of comprehensive traditional home care programs. Gerontologist, 26(4): 382-388.

This article discusses the fact that the clientele of these two types of home care programs--the comprehensive and the traditional--are similar, and that clients in the comprehensive programs neither have more problems nor less social supports than those in traditional programs, as is sometimes asserted. The areas of highest need in both types of programs were identified as homemaker and personal care services. Valuable resource for administrators of home care programs and care providers.

226. Benefield L. E. (ed.) (1988). Home Health Care Management. Englewood Cliffs, NJ: Prentice Hall.

Topics discussed by many experts include trends in home health care, legal aspects of home health management, financial management, management information systems, staffing structure, quality assurance, marketing, diversification and restructuring, personnel issues, productivity, roles of staff and supervisors, and kinds of treatment in different health care settings. The content, organization, and scope of this book are excellent, making it a valuable reference for administrators in home health care.

227. Beuscher T. L. (1991). The CNS: A valuable resource in home care. Caring, 10(4):22-25.

Nurses with advanced education and clinical expertise are increasingly needed in the homecare setting to provide high tech care. The master's prepared clinical nurse specialist (CNS) is one example of an experienced nurse who can function effectively within the interdisciplinary health care team. In addition to nursing skills, nurses with master's degrees also have administration, education, and research knowledge and experience, so that the CNS or nurse practitioner (NP) can fill a variety of roles.

228. Crystal S., Flemming C., Beck P., Smolka G. (1987). The Management of Home Care Services. New York: Springer Publishing Company.

This book is a revision and extension of the final report of the Home Care Fiscal Management Project, funded by a Department of Health and Human Services grant through the Administration on Aging. The project's purpose was to identify innovative public fiscal management practices in home care and to provide access to information on these practices to those who either offer or contract for home care services. Sections include an overview of the home care system, fiscal management, personnel practices, and others, with application of these areas to specific local and state programs.

229. DeGraff A. H. (1988). Home Health Aides. Clifton Park, NY: Saratoga Access Publications.

Management skills, strategies for being a good manager, types of help and services that each provides, identifying individual needs, salaries and taxes, recruiting, interviewing, training, and parting with help are the topics covered in this detailed manual for administrators in home care agencies.

230. Department of Aging, New York City (1984). Delivery of Medical and Social Services to the Homebound Elderly: A Demonstration of Intersystem Coordination. Washington, DC: Policy Information Center, ID# 3542.

This project's overall purpose was to test a community-based approach to the delivery of medical and social services to 635 homebound, chronically ill elderly who were Medicare Part B eligible and living in New York City between 1980 and 1984. The goal was to enable the participants to remain out of institutional settings by providing appropriate enabling services. Findings showed that a strong need exists among this population for these services and that a relatively limited expansion of home care benefits to this population could be successful in achieving the desired goal.

231. Dunkle R. E., Wykle M. L. (1988). Decision Making in Long-Term Care: Factors in Planning. New York: Springer Publishing Company.

This is a report based on a symposium sponsored by Case Western Reserve University's Center on Aging and Health, November 1986. The purpose of the conference was to assist in improving professional performance in decision making regarding extended care of older people. The book is divided into four major sections: 1) health care policy and ethical concerns, 2) psychosocial perspec--tives, 3) legal parameters, and 4) costs. It provides various views on the causes and consequences of decision making but little regarding their interrelationships.

232. Dychtwald K., Zitter M., Levison J. (1990). Implementing Eldercare Services: Strategies That Work. New York: McGraw-Hill.

The many varieties of home or eldercare services are explored and advocated as a means of decreasing health care costs for the increasing number of older persons. The kind of services provided depends on the individual's situation and needs, and includes adult day care, homemaker services, respite care, Meals on Wheels, etc. A forceful argument is presented in favor of these kinds of services to permit the elderly access to needed services that are appropriate for a particular time in life. Recommended for home health care agency administrators, families, and providers of services.

233. Fashimpar G (1983). A management tool for evaluating the adequacy and quality of homemaker-home health aide programs. Gerontologist, 23(2):127-131.

This article reports on the testing of a Homemaker and Home Health Aide Program Evaluation Questionnaire which was found to be valid, reliable, and relatively inexpensive. The evaluation addresses homemaker/client relationships, job performance, and achievement of objectives in a sample of 40 clients. The tool can be used for overall program evaluation, as well as for individual performance and to assess relationships between caregivers and clients. Recommended for home care agency administrators and quality assurance team members.

234. Feldman P. H. (1988). The Impact and Feasibility

of Efforts to Reduce Turnover in the Home Care Industry. ERIC, # ED 320066.

This paper describes a Ford Foundation demonstration project for improving the quality of work life and reducing turnover with homemakers/home health aides. The project modified training and support, pay and benefits, status, opportunities for advancement, and hours of work. Eighteen months after these interventions those who received them were 21-44% more likely to have remained on the job than subjects in a control group.

235. Feldman P. H. (1988). Understanding Job Satisfaction and Turnover in the Home Aide Work Force. ERIC document # ED 320065.

This paper describes a model that was developed to explain job satisfaction and turnover in home health aides. This model was tested with survey data from a home care demonstration project that was supported by the Ford Foundation. Job satisfaction was seen to be influenced by positive attitudes about pay and benefits, supervisor supportiveness, and task variety. Factors that determined intent to leave were youth, loneliness, and dissatisfaction with pay and benefits.

236. Feldman P. H., Sapienza A. M., Kane N. M. (1990). Who Cares for Them? Workers in the Home Health Care Industry. Westport, CT: Greenwood Press.

This substantive resource includes four parts: the labor market, case studies of the work life demonstrations, overview of work life programs, and recommendations and policy implications. The objectives of the book were fully addressed: 1) to identify critical factors affecting the working conditions and job satisfaction of the home aide work force, 2) to assess the feasibility of and evaluate the impact of changes designed to improve work life of home aides, and 3) to develop implications for administrators and policy planners in the home health care arena.

237. General Accounting Office (1990). Posthospital

Care: Discharge Planners Report Increasing Difficulty in Placing Medicare Patients. Washington, DC: Policy Information Center, ID# 2828.

The results of a survey of hospital discharge planners is reported regarding their perceptions of problems placing Medicare patients in skilled nursing facilities or in home health care services post-hospital discharge. Of those surveyed, 97% reported difficulty in skilled nursing home placement, while 86% reported difficulty with home health care placement. The greatest barrier to placement in either care system were the rules and regulations governing Medicare. The implementation of the prospective payment system was considered to have the greatest negative impact on post-hospital placement during the 1982-1985 period. The recent increase in the number of home health agencies was seen as facilitating access.

238. Giardina C. W., Fottler M. D., Shewchuk R. M., Hill D. B. (1990). The case for hospital diversification into long-term care. Health Care Management Review, 15(1):71-82.

Because the market for long-term care (LTC) services is expected to grow rapidly in the years ahead, the case for hospital diversification into LTC is a strong one. Among the areas of LTC that hospitals will manage are home health care agencies. There are distinct advantages for both the hospital and clients as a result of this integrated system: hospitals will become more responsive to clients' needs, there is expected to be mutual commitment of the institution and the client, and the allegation that the hospital is "dumping" patients without providing an avenue for continuity of care is nullified.

239. Griffith D. (1986). Blending key ingredients to assure quality in home health care. Nursing and Health Care, 7(6):301-302.

This article describes strategies that home care agencies can use to improve their services. Among these strategies are careful staff selection, appropriate and timely training, and evaluation of aspects of the situation. Measures of the quality of care are provided, including accreditation standards and procedures. Excellent resource for administrators of home health care agencies.

240. Igoe J. F., Hawkins J. W., Johnson E. E., Utley Q. E. (1989). Nurse-managed approach to care. Geriatr Nurs, 10(1):32-34.

Nurse practitioner faculty began and operated a nurse-managed center for three years. Clients were primarily older persons who visited their regular physicians once a year, then sought continuing care from NPs in the center. Cost was half that charged by other health professionals, and client satisfaction was high. The group emphasized the need for more such centers.

241. Jamieson M., Martinson I. (1983). Block nursing: Neighbors caring for neighbors. Nursing Outlook, 31(5):270, 272-273.

The authors describe a program in St. Paul, Minnesota in which nursing care is delivered to neighbors, by neighbors, to allow older people to remain independent and at home. Health education, disease prevention, and health maintenance are stressed as important factors for maintaining people in their homes. This activity can be used as a model by other communities. Recommended for health care planners, community agencies, and caregivers for the elderly.

242. Kirschner C., Rosengarten L. (1982). The skilled social work role in home care. Social Work, 27(6):527-529.

This article describes the specialized, skilled roles that social workers have in the home health care system. It defines how social workers can work within an interdisciplinary framework using both separate and collaborative relationships with the home care team. Recommended resource for home care agency administrators, social workers, caregivers, and others providing or coordinating home care services.

243. Kosberg J., Cairl R. (1986). The cost of care index: A case management tool for screening care providers. Gerontologist, 26(3):273-278.

The Cost of Care Index (CCI) is presented in this article. It is a 20-item case management tool that focuses on five dimensions related to family care of elderly persons. The Index is used to assess families and to identify actual and perceived problems in families caring for elderly relatives. This assessment tool can be a valuable resource for home care administrators and care providers.

244. Mebane M. L. (1991). Designing a clinical career ladder for the home care nurse. Caring, 10(4):16-20.

Because nurses are needed in every setting and are rewarded at high levels in some settings, they have a choice of selecting the situation or position that promotes the greatest advantages and incentives. Home care agencies must compete for nurses as well, and administrators need to creatively develop strategies that will provide opportunities for home care nurses to advance. One such incentive is that of career ladder with established criteria which are clear and will ensure that nurses can advance steadily within the system.

245. Meisenheimer C. G. (1989). Quality Assurance for Home Health Care. Rockville, MD: Aspen Publishers, Inc.

The author provides a valuable resource book which encompasses topic areas such as historical background and future implications of home health care; quality assurance process; standards of quality assurance; problem identification, monitoring, and evaluation; data collection methods; documentation; perspectives from physicians, nurses, social workers, and therapists; practice issues; legal and ethical issues; caregivers; and examples of existing high-quality home health agencies.

246. Miller J. A. (1991). Community-Based Long-Term Care: Innovative Models. Newbury Park, CA: Sage Publications.

This book provides detailed and factual information about 12 community-based health care programs that are successfully meeting the needs of elderly clients in their communities. The information will be of benefit to anyone concerned with trying to build better systems of care delivery for our growing elderly population who reside outside of institutional settings.

247. National Council on Aging (1990). Senior Center Standards. National Council on Aging, Department 5087, Washington, DC 20061-5087.

This publication describes the new challenges and broader mission that senior centers face in the 1990s because of the increasingly complex environment in which senior centers operate. Senior centers serve a rapidly growing population of well and frail elderly, and must reach out to the underserved, low-income, and minority elderly groups, provide information and access to services and referrals for those who need them, raise and manage funds from many sources, and be responsive to a broad range of community needs. Highly recommended for administrators, health care professionals, and policy planners.

248. National Leadership Commission on Health Care (U.S.) (1989). For the Health of a Nation: A Shared Responsibility. Ann Arbor, MI: Health Administration Press.

This commission report is based upon a request to provide information concerning realistic solutions to the problems of excessive health care costs, barriers to access, and quality assurance/risk management issues. Probable solutions to these issues are provided and additional information is reported regarding proposals for reforming the medical professional liability system and for developing national health care guidelines.

249. O'Brien B. M. (1991). Implementing a pay-per-visit program while ensuring quality care. Caring, 10(4):26-28.

Developing creative staffing alternatives that meet quality assurance standards and that respond to current market trends is one of the challenges facing home care administrators today. One plan to increase productivity and cost-effectiveness of home care was implemented in a Passaic, NJ program. The program included a quality assurance reporting structure that greatly facilitated communications and documentation. Results of the plan were a drop in turnover rate among staff, a return of some staff who had previously left, and a 17% increase in visit volume.

250. Peters D. A., Eigsti D. M. (1991). In search of excellence: The personnel issue of the future. Caring, 10(4):12-14.

Deming's principle of total quality management is appropriate and applicable to the home care setting with respect to formulating, implementing and evaluating quality of care. Quality care is contingent on competent staff empowered to carry out their roles in an environment that recognizes and rewards personal excellence.

251. Saba V., O'Hare P. A. et al (1991). A nursing intervention taxonomy for home health care. Nursing & Health Care, 12(6):296-299.

The authors describe a method for classifying home health Medicare patients to predict resource requirements and to measure outcomes of home care provided. The taxonomy is useful for home care agencies because it can also be used to structure reimbursement for care providers. Helpful nursing interventions and their implications for further development of home care practice, research, and policy.

252. Schwartz P. J., Blumenfield S., Simon E. P. (1990). The interim homecare program: An innovative discharge planning alternative. Health and Social Work,

15(2):152-160.

Because hospitals are under increasing pressure to discharge patients as soon as possible, many patients require additional time to recover physically, emotionally, financially, and socially. The Interim Homecare Project (IHP) developed at Mount Sinai Medical Center's Department of Social Work Services provides time-limited intensive home health care aide services for elderly patients who are at risk of lengthened recovery times. IHP patients had shortened length of stay, with the shorter stay exceeding expectations and estimates based on comparison groups.

253. Smith M. J. (1990). Program Evaluation in the Human Services. New York: Springer Publishing Company.

This text provides a comprehensive introduction to evaluating human services. The "how-to" format shows the whole process of program evaluation from beginning to end using explicit examples. Topics included are descriptions of programs, defining program goals, amd designing evaluation studies. Aspects of program implementation, evaluation, and data analysis are discussed. Case studies and exercises allow for application of principles and methods presented.

254. Sullivan H. K. (1991). An incentive plan for nurses: Linking bonuses to both care and documentation. Caring, 10(4):26-28.

Quality care does not equate with level of productivity; both are necessary in the home care setting. This article focuses on ways to develop incentive bonus programs to recruit and retain highly qualified and committed home care staff. Part of the methodology to measure quality is to evaluate the documentation that states that care has been provided. Standards must be in place against which individuals are tested.

255. Vinton L. (1991). Health-care connections: Linking hospital and community-based care for the elderly and their caregivers. Gerontology and Geriatrics Education,

<u>11</u>(3):57-66.

Due to Medicare cost containment strategies, older persons are being hospitalized for shorter periods, and have greater care needs on discharge, which require continuity of care. This article focuses on a joint project developed by an acute care hospital and a community care agency to effect formal linkages between systems in order to provide care to both elders and their caregivers, often family members. Results of the project include a resource guide to community-based services, a training curriculum, and an implementation plan.

256. White J. L. (1991). The health care nursing shortage: Increased demand and recommended action. <u>Caring</u>, <u>10</u>(4):4-6.

In its sixth year, the current nursing shortage is the most persistent and prolonged shortage of nurses that the country has experienced. The causes are multifactorial, but the most significant factors is the rapid and continuing increase in demand for nursing services. Skilled nurses are particularly needed to provide high tech home care, and this need will continue to grow. The expertise of nurse practitioners has also become more fully recognized in both acute and long-term care settings. All segments of the federal, state, and local governments will need to provide policies to facilitate further increases in the supply of registered nurses.

257. Williams S. D., Williams J. R. (1988). <u>How to Market Home Health Care Services</u>. New York: John Wiley & Sons.

Between 1978 and 1986 the number of hospital-based home health care agencies more than doubled to over 1000, and the number of independent agencies increased by 80%. While home health care is growing, many clients do not perceive the need for or the availability of these services. The authors say that marketing provides a client-centered focus that forces organizations to identify and meet clients' needs. The book's four parts include a general discussion of marketing, traditional marketing concepts, creation and implementation of a marketing plan. The final section addresses ethical issues in marketing, and the potential future markets for home health care agencies. Comprehensive resource for administrators and marketing managers.

258. Yeatts D. E. et al (1987). Evaluation of Connecticut's Medicaid community care waiver program. Gerontologist, 27(5):652-659.

This Connecticut program provided resources for elderly persons to participate in home and community-based services, rather than enter a nursing home. The authors support careful screening of applicants to programs to assure appropriate identification of the population to be serviced. Cost effectiveness of the program was not conclusive. This article presents an overview of how one community met the challenges of the elderly population and their needs.

6

Research

259. Abbott Northwestern Hospital (1987). Study of Factors That Promote Home Health Care of Older Persons, 2 volumes. Washington, DC: Policy Information Center, PIC ID# 3472.

The role of family members in providing informal home care services to frail and chronically ill elderly relatives was determined and the impact of formal support systems on the promotion of home care was assessed. A total of 457 primary family caregivers were interviewed as part of the data collection process. Findings concluded that family members provided the vast majority of services needed by their relatives and were intensively involved in every aspect of care. Few formal services were utilized and those that were included homemakers and visitation. The most commonly used community-based services were day care centers and senior centers.

260. Administration on Aging (1991). Determining the Impact of Gerontology Preparation on Personnel in the Aging Network. Washington, DC: Association for Gerontology in Higher Education.

This Federally funded study, conducted by the University of Southern California (USC) and the Association for Gerontology in Higher Education (AGHE), examines the characteristics of jobs and professional employees in the aging network. During three months in 1990, 3200 questionnaires were sent to all professionals whose job required a knowledge of aging who were employed by State Units on Aging (SUA) and to a random sample of professionals employed in the 120 Area Agencies on Aging (AAA). Consistent with the functions of the SUAs and AAAs defined in the 1973 Amendments to the Older Americans Act, professionals were defined as persons whose primary responsibilities were to plan, evaluate, coordinate, broker, or administer programs or services on behalf of the Agency or older Americans, or who provided direct care to aging persons. The final report summarizing survey data from 1316 SUA and 813 AAA respondents is available from the AGHE, 1001 Connecticut Avenue, NW, Suite 410, Washington, DC 20036-5504, or call 202/429-9277.

261. Alderman A. (1990). Social Services for the Elderly: The Relationship Between Title III of the Older Americans Act and the Social Services Block Grant (Phase I). Washington, DC: Policy Information Center, PIC ID# 3357.

This is the first of a series of three phases studying the social services provided to the elderly. This study examined the complex relationships at the state and local levels involved in administering two federal programs, i.e., Social Services Block Grants administered by the state social service agencies, and the Older Americans Act administered by the state units on aging. This report provides information gathered from a total of 52 states. Highly recommended for social service workers and administrators, policy planners, providers, and researchers.

262. Archbold P. G., Stewart B. J., Greenlick M. R., Harvath T. (1990). Mutuality and preparedness as predictors of caregiver role strain. Res Nurs & Health, 13(6):375-384.

The researchers studied factors that relate to role strain among family caregivers of older persons recently discharged home from hospital. Mutuality (caregiver's ability to feel gratified in the situation), and preparedness (caregiver's perception of self as capable) were significant factors in ameliorating but not eliminating all role strain.

263. Baillie V., Norbeck J. S., Barnes L. E. (1988). Stress, social support, and psychological distress of family caregivers of the elderly. Nurs Res, 37(4):217-222.

The effects of stress and social support and their interaction with the psychological well-being of 87 family caregivers of impaired elderly were examined. Perceived stress and satisfaction with support accounted for 32%-36% of variance in psychological distress or depression. The findings indicate that caregivers who are caring for a mentally impaired elderly, who have been providing care for an extended time, and who have low social support, are at high risk for psychological distress or depression.

264. Birren J., Schaie W. K. (1990). Handbook of the Psychology of Aging, 3rd Edition. San Diego, CA: Academic Press.

The two previous editions came to be seen as the definitive reference source for information about the psychology of adult development and aging. This new edition reviews recent developments in research on such topics as social and biological influence on behavior, cognitive functions in the elderly individual, and animal models in aging. New topics include: 1) Concepts of time in aging, 2) Creativity and wisdom, 3) Human factors, and 4) Ethics in research on aging.

265. Brody B. A. (ed.) (1989). Suicide and Euthanasia: Historical and Contemporary Themes. Boston: Kluwer Academic Publishers.

Suicide and euthanasia are discussed by seven ethics philosophers in the context of historical philosophy. Reformation and Renaissance scholars, early Christians and Jews, and Greek philosophers are among those whose views are presented. Thought-provoking reading for all health care professionals, administrators, and policy planners.

266. Brown F. (1986). Research Agenda for Evaluating the Impact of PPS on Long-Term Care. Washington, DC: Policy Information Center, ID# 2410.

Five major gaps are identified for research in the existing knowledge of the impact of the Medicare prospective payment system on care for frail elderly and individuals with acute underlying medical conditions. The policy relevance of each of the following gaps is discussed: 1) patterns of experience post-discharge, 2) discharge planning process, 3) home health care, 4) nursing home care, and 5) hospital readmission. Excellent background on these topics that is applicable in current delivery systems.

267. Bush M. (1989). Community Care for the Elderly: An International Perspective. Washington, DC: Policy Information Center, ID# 3366.

Home care services were examined in Great Britain, the Netherlands, Norway, Sweden, Canada, Manitoba, and Argentina to determine how prominent service issues for the elderly in this country were being dealt with in these other countries. Numerous findings are presented in this Final Report. Significant among them is the fact that all these countries have a specific government policy toward home care that recognizes it as a viable and essential program for long-term care.

268. Deeg D. J. H. (1989). Experiences from Longitudinal Studies of Aging. Nijmegen, The Netherlands: Netherlands Institute of Gerontology.

While the need for longitudinal research is evident, the associated problems in conducting this type of study are frequently underestimated. Such problems can arise in the methodology, organization, administration, financing, substantive theory, and interpretation and generalizability of findings. This book provides cumulative information to assist researchers to conduct longitudinal research more effectively by avoiding many of the inherent pitfalls.

269. Doty P. (1989). Caregiver Burden and Institutionalization, Hospital Use and Stability of Care. Washington, DC: Policy Information Center, ID# 3334.

Researchers examined the effect of "caregiving burden" on nursing home admission, hospital use, and stability of the family and professional care network. Data from the 1982-84 National Long Term Care Survey and the Informal Caregivers Survey are included in this report. Results of the study and recommendations are presented.

270. Dwyer J. W., Seccombe K. (1991). Elder care as family labor: The influence of gender and family position. J Fam Issues, 12(2):229.

This research shows that gender differences in the performance of specific caregiving tasks and the amount of time spent providing care by family caregivers of frail elderly should be considered in the context of family position-related patterns and expectations. Using a sample of 813 impaired elderly people and their caregivers, researchers found that husbands (as compared with wives) and daughters (as compared with sons) report spending more time and performing a greater number of caregiving tasks. The factor of family position may confound interpretations about the relationship between gender and family caregiving.

271. Ellingson K. (1989). Nursing Home Without Walls: Evaluation of the New York State Long-Term Home Health Care Program. Washington, DC: Policy Information Center, ID# 1854.

This research demonstration project provided skilled nursing home level of care to patients in their homes in New York state. Its chief purpose was to determine whether this could be a viable alternative to nursing home care in terms of cost, utilization, and effectiveness. Outcomes revealed that urban center costs exceeded those of upstate client costs and that across the entire state, services could have been more cost-effective if subsets of clients were targeted for whom long-term home health care is most cost effective. Levels of nursing home utilization by these clients were reduced across all sites in the study. Recommended for administrators of home health care agencies, nursing homes, and policy planners.

272. Funk S. G., Tornquist E. M. et al (1990). Key Aspects of Recovery: Improving Nutrition, Rest, and Mobility. New York: Springer Publishing Company.

This book is the result of a research grant awarded to the School of Nursing, University of North Carolina at Chapel Hill by the National Center for Nursing Research to disseminate knowledge resulting from nursing research and demonstration projects. Chapters are written by nurse experts in the field, and address infant nutrition, rest, and mobility; adult nutrition, skin integrity, rest, mobility, and recovery. Valuable fund of information based on substantial research.

273. Gibson R. C. (1991). Age-by-race differences in health and functioning of elderly persons. J Aging & Health, 3(3):335-351.

Health data on the elderly population showed four trends: 1) a younger Black group that was more morbid than an older Black group, 2) an alternating pattern of Black morbid and robust age groups, 3) a Black disadvantage in health and functioning that was greater in race comparisons involving the Black morbid and less in comparisons involving the Black robust age groups, and 4) a Black health detriment that seemed to narrow at age 85. These trends indicate that age and health are more strongly correlated in the White elderly than in the Black elderly.

274. Goldstein A. A. (1990). Data base news in aging: Interagency forum on aging-related statistics. Federal Forum. Washington, DC: Population Division, Bureau of the Census.

The purpose of this information bulletin is to bring news of recent development in databases of interest to researchers and others in the field of aging. The bulletin is published periodically and all Federal agencies are invited to participate.

275. Graber G., Thomasma D. (1990). Euthanasia: Toward an Ethical Social Policy. New York: Continuum Press.

The authors develop a premise that today, there is little need for active euthanasia if more attention is paid to controlling pain and suffering, and to the patient's value system. If providers can give more specific responses to patients' requests to die, and if plans are made with the patient's family about the best way to bring about a kind and merciful death, the issue can be resolved well for all concerned. A problem arises only when the system does not work properly. Many perspectives are included for the purpose of presenting all sides to this controversial area, to allow reasoned and logical decisions to be made in a timely way.

276. Graveley E. A., Oseasohn C. S. (1991). Multiple drug regimens: medication compliance among veterans 65 years and older. Res Nurs & Health, 14(1):51-58.

This study identified compliant/noncompliant male veterans. Data showed only two significant factors: ethnicity and number of daily prescribed pills. Interviews revealed common problems: physician changing medication or dosage and client not knowing, forgetting to reorder drugs, difficulty in breaking tablets when 1/2 was prescribed, and similar kinds of barriers to compliance.

277. Gubrium J. F. (1989). The domestic meaning of institutionalization. In Research on Adulthood and Aging: The Human Science Approach. L. E. Thomas (ed.) Albany: State University of New York Press, 90-104.

Recent research findings about many aspects of aging are relevant to health professionals in home care and caregivers to help them understand the physiological and psychological changes that occur with aging. Gubrium's chapter discusses making the decision between whether to continue caring for the elderly member(s) in the home or to choose a nursing home with a "homey" environment.

278. Guralnik J. M., LaCroix A. Z., Branch L. G., Kasl S. V., Wallace R. B. (1991). Morbidity and disability in older persons in the years prior to death. Amer J Publ Health, 81:443-447.

This study examined chronic conditions and disability of three community-based cohorts of persons age 65 and older (N = 531) for 3 years prior to death. The subjects received 3 annual physical assessments and then died within one year of the third assessment. The number of chronic conditions, prevalence of disability in activities of daily living (ADLs), and prevalence of disability on a modified Rosow-Breslau scale were determined for the decedents, and compared to 8821 members of the cohorts known to have survived. The results have important implications for disability levels in future older populations in which death is projected to occur at increasingly higher ages.

279. Hall M. (1981). Measuring Geriatric Home Care Utilization, Effects, and Costs. Washington, DC: Policy Information Center, NTIS No. PB 84-139443; ID# 3514.

Records of over 2000 older adults served by the San Francisco Home Health Services, Inc. (1968-75) were analyzed to identify relationships between client characteristics beginning home health care and utilization patterns and client status at time of discharge. Major findings include that pay plans were the predominant predictor of the intensity of services received and Medicare clients used services more intensively than others, while Medicaid clients averaged a longer duration of home care with less intensity than other clients. Much of this information is useful over time. Recommended for administrators of home health care agencies, policy planners, and researchers.

280. Hall M. (1986). Study of Home Respiratory Therapy:

Report to Congress. Washington, DC: Policy Information Center, ID# 2184.

The state of the art in respiratory therapy and its availability as a covered home health care benefit for Medicare clients is the topic, developed by the Health Care Financing Administration (HCFA) at the request of Congress. The report recommends that respiratory therapy services be retained as a benefit, and that these services do not need to be expanded because they are adequate if the system is running well. Basic reimbursement for most home health care services is proposed.

281. Hedrick S. C., Koepsell T. D., Inui T. (1989). Meta-analysis of home-care effects on mortality and nursing home placement. Med Care, 27(11):1015-26.

This meta-analysis was designed to show how the relatively new discipline of meta-analysis can be employed in health services research. The results of 13 studies of the effect of home care on mortality and nursing home placement were examined using this methodology. Analysis showed that there was a small, beneficial effect of home care on mortality, but was not statistically significant. There was stronger evidence of reduction in nursing home placements. One outcome was the determination that log-linear modeling made it easier to detect and explore study-to-study variation in home care effects.

282. Hickey E. (1987). Assessment of the Current Utilization of Community Migrant Health Centers by the Elderly. Washington, DC: Policy Information Center, PIC ID# 2852.

This study provides the Bureau of Health Care Delivery and Assistance the basis for making policy decisions regarding health care delivery to the elderly. A model of care was developed by this study, and BHCDA recommended that all CMHCs use this for their geriatric service provision. The model includes a team approach to care, presenting a broad range of services utilizing financially sound third-party payor contracts and increasing collaborative relationships to strengthen aging and other health and social service provisions.

283. Husaini B. A., Moore S. T. (1991). Arthritis disability, depression, and life satisfaction among black elderly people. Health & Soc Work, 15(4):253-260.

This study examined the correlates of arthritis disorder in a sample of black elderly people in Nashville, Tennessee. Both the presence of arthritis and its severity were studied in relation to the level of depression and life satisfaction in the areas of family life, social support, and leisure activities. Findings showed that arthritic black elderly people were more depressed and experienced lower levels of life satisfaction than nonarthritic black elderly people.

284. Lewis M.A., Leake B., Clark V., Leal-Sotelo M. (1989). Case mix and outcomes of nursing home patients. The importance of prior nursing home care and admission from home versus hospital. Medical Care, 27(4):376-385.

The researchers compared the personal characteristics, measures of functional status/case mix, and discharge outcomes of nursing home patients admitted to skilled nursing facilities (SNFs) in 1984 for the first time (first admission) to those of patients with a prior history of nursing home care (readmissions). Readmitted patients were more disabled and debilitated, significantly less likely to return home, and more likely to be hospitalized. The conclusion is that history of prior nursing home admission(s) is an important indicator of prognosis, service needs, length of stay of patients in the nursing home, and their discharge outcomes. Location before admission--home versus hospital--was associated with case mix descriptors, and length of stay was unrelated to discharge outcomes.

285. Mangano M. (1978). Home Health Care: A Service Delivery Assessment. Washington, DC: Policy Information Center, ID# 2335.

An assessment is provided of in-home services to the elderly through Medicare, Medicaid and Social Services programs. Findings include: 1) multiply impaired elderly were the major recipients of services, 2) service availability is not well known, 3) clients play a passive role, 4) service delivery is uncoordinated, 5) providers preferred serving Medicare clientele, and 6) administrative problems inhibited cost-effective service delivery. Excellent background information about these topics primarily for researchers.

286. Mangano M. (1981). Medicare Home Health Services: A Service Delivery Assessment (three reports). Washington, DC: Policy Information Center, ID# 2294.

This study's purpose was to determine the extent and type of changes taking place among Medicare certified home health providers, and how clients gain access to these and other services. Major findings showed that 1) competition is prevalent, 2) sick and elderly clients comprise the majority served, 3) nurses function as the gatekeepers to services, 4) hospital discharge planning is limited, and 5) assessment and referral practices are more comprehensive than that of hospitals. Two additional reports are: Competition: An Emerging Force in a Changing Home Health Field, and Changing Patterns of Entry to Home Health Services. Substantive background information for administrators, care providers, and researchers in this field.

287. McCorkle R., Benoliel J. Q., Donaldson G., Georgiadou F. et al (1989). A randomized clinical trial of home nursing care for lung cancer patients. Cancer, 64(6):1375-82.

This clinical trial was conducted to assess the effects of home nursing care for patients with progressive lung cancer. The sample included 166 patients who were assigned either to an oncology home care group (OHC) that received care from oncology home care nurses, a standard home care group (SHC) that received care from regular home care nurses, or an office care group (OC) that received whatever care they needed except for home care. The patients were admitted to the study group 2 months after diagnosis, and followed for 6 months. The two home care groups had less distress and greater independence 6 weeks longer than the office care group.

288. Mishra S. I., Aldwin C. M., Colby B. N., Oseas R. S. (1991). Adaptive potential stress and natural killer cell activity in older adults. J Aging & Health, 3(3): 368-387.

The researchers examined the relationship among psychosocial vulnerability (stress) and resilience (adaptive potential) factors and three outcome measures: self-reported physical symptoms, positive and negative affect, and natural killer cell activity in 39 male and female older adults residing in a retirement community (mean age was 73.5 years). Although life events were directly related to physical symptoms, both perceived that stress and adaptive potential were significantly associated with positive and negative affect. There was a tendency for adaptive potential to buffer the effect of perceived stress on negative affect. However, natural killer cell activity was not significantly related to any psychosocial vulnerability and resilience factors in this small sample.

289. Moore F. M. (1988). Homemaker-Home Health Aide Services. Owings Mills, MD: National Health Publishing.

This book presents a comprehensive review of home health care and the use of aides in providing care. Topics addressed include type of care available, payment sources, coordination of services, and quality of services. Also examined are programs of care available in other countries, which are contrasted with care in the U.S. Recommended for administrators of home health care agencies, providers, clients, and families.

290. Mor-Barak M. E., Miller L. S., Syme L. S. (1991). Social networks, life events, and health of the poor, frail elderly: a longitudinal study of the buffering versus the direct effect. Fam Community Health, 14(2): 1-13.

Research over the past twenty years has established both a theoretical basis and empirical evidence for the relationship between social ties and health. This research examined the causal link between social network, life events, and the poor, frail elderly. The sample was derived from data collected on 3559 poor, frail elderly, each of whom had two to four assessments. The individuals were participants in the California Multipurpose Senior Services Project (MSSP). The study sought to determine whether data supported the "buffering hypothesis," which suggests that social relationships can combat ill health that often results from stressful life events. Findings were that social networks are significant predictors of self-rated health in the short term, but not in the long term.

291. National Institutes of Health (1989). Older and wiser. The Baltimore Longitudinal Study of Aging. NIH Publication no. 89-2797, September.

This study provides a description of some of the major research themes and findings related to aging. The report is based on writings and interviews with BLSA scientist and research participants in this, the longest running scientific examination of human aging.

292. Nugent D. (1987). AFDC Homemaker-Home Health Aide Demonstration: Overview of Evaluation Results. Washington, DC: Policy Information Center, ID# 2157.

A demonstration project was mandated by Congress whereby AFDC recipients were to be trained in care of the elderly and disabled to prevent institutionalization and to reduce welfare dependency. Seven states were included in the study and a cost-benefit analysis was conducted. Numerous data collection instruments were developed and secondary data sources included Medicaid, SSI. AFDC, Medicare, and the Food Stamp Program.

293. Oktay J. S., Palley H. A. (1991). The Medicaid personal care services program: Implications for social work practice. Health & Social Work, 16(2):110-114.

Results of a survey of Medicaid personal care programs in 15 states and the District of Columbia in 1987 showed that these programs have multiple internal problems which detract from their efficiency and effectiveness. Among the problems identified were: low wages, delayed payment, lack of coordination among agencies, lack of standards for training and supervising workers, unequal access to programs, and inequities among states. The result is that the programs have difficulty recruiting and retaining qualified workers. This study has implications for social workers as well as other members of the community and home health care teams.

294. Ory M. G., Abeles R. P. (1991). Aging, Health, and Behavior. Newbury Park, CA: Sage Publications.

A presentation of basic and applied research on aging, health, and behavior, drawn from both American and European experiences. Contributors explore the influence of age and ethnicity on health and behavior, coping with chronic illness and disability, the effects of stress on illness, disease prevention, and health promotion, and the implications for public policy.

295. Pasquale D. K. (1988). Characteristics of Medicare-eligible home care clients. Public Health Nurs, 5(3):129-34.

Providers, consumers, and legislators seem to agree that today's home care population is older and sicker. Little information exists that describes the characteristics of this population. Retrospective review of 100 randomly selected clinical records from a large not-for-profit home care agency yielded data. Findings revealed that chronic health care problems predominated, that over half of the sample had at least moderate functional impairment, that female recipients tended to be older and rely on informal caregivers, that females were usually more functionally impaired than males, and that wives usually provided care to male clients. The major conclusion was that the Medicare home care population is not homogeneous, but is a diverse group that likely has age and gender variants.

296. Polinsky M. L., Fred C., Ganz P. A. (1991). Quantitative and qualitative assessment of a case management program for cancer patients. Health & Soc Work, 16(3):176-183.

An oncology social work case management model of intervention is described quantitatively and qualitatively. Sixty-nine newly diagnosed breast cancer patients followed by telephone for one year required 374 hours of the social worker's time in providing reassurance, information, and referral to existing community resources. This telephone-based model was found to be highly effective and cost-effective in addressing the rehabilitation needs of cancer patients.

297. Reed P. G. (1991). Self-transcendence and mental health in oldest-old adults. Nurs Res, 40(1):5-11.

A study of 55 independent-living adults, aged 80 to 97, showed that a significant inverse relationship exists between self-transcendence and symptoms such as depression, thus demonstrating the importance of expansion of self boundaries in older persons.

298. Roos N. P., Havens M. A. (1991). Predictors of successful aging: A twelve-year study of Manitoba elderly. Amer J Publ Health, 81(1):63-68.

In Canada, a representative cohort of elderly individuals aged 65-84 (N = 3573) were interviewed in 1971, and the survivors were interviewed again in 1983. The analysis assessed the determinants of successful aging--whether or not an individual will live to an advanced age, continue to function well at home, and remain mentally alert. Those who aged successfully were shown to have greater satisfaction with life in 1983 and to have made fewer demands on the health care sytem than those who aged less well. Of the many variables examined, only four measures of health status, two measures of mental status, and not having one's spouse die or enter a nursing home were shown to be predictive of successful aging.

299. Shapiro E., Roos N. (1989). Predictors and patterns of nursing home and home care use. In Health Care of the Elderly. M. D. Petersen, D. L. White (eds.). Newbury Park, CA: Sage Publications, 127-166.

This chapter presents a review of the literature on predictors of nursing home use and home care use, patterns of nursing home and home care use, the impact of nursing home residency on hospital use, and cohort effects on the use of nursing home and home care services. Predictors of patterns of use of these services emerge from the findings. Recommended for administrators of nursing homes and home care agencies, providers of care in these settings, and researchers.

300. Shapiro E., Tate E. B. (1989). Is health care changing? A comparison between physician, hospital, nursing home, and home care use of two elderly cohorts. Med Care, 27(11):1002-14.

This study used log-linear survival analysis and log-rank tests to compare 1) characteristics of two elderly cohorts (1971 and 1976), 2) their use of physician, hospital, nursing home and home care services over 8.5 years, and 3) physician and bed supplies during the two periods. Both cohorts were similar in health status and in their use of hospital, nursing home, and home care resources despite a steady decrease in available hospital and nursing home beds during the period. The later cohort used significantly more ambulatory care than the earlier group.

301. Silverman P. (ed.) (1988). The Elderly as Modern Pioneers. Bloomington, IL: Indiana University Press.

A summary of gerontological research is presented from an anthropological perspective. A good reference book for all who work with the elderly. A multidisciplinary and transcultural approach is utilized in presenting the information. Recommended particularly for gerontological faculty, researchers, administrators, and policy planners.

302. Speake D. L., Cowart M. E., Stephens R. (1991). Healthy lifestyle practices of rural and urban elderly. Health Values, 15(1):45-56.

Research studies show that adopting healthy lifestyle practices may prevent or slow the physical decline of, and promote well-being in, the elderly. Data indicate that health status of the rural elderly is worse than that of their urban counterparts. Six lifestyle practices were examined in comparing the two groups: stress management, exercise, nutrition, health responsibility, self-actualization, and interpersonal support. Survey data from 343 volunteer elderly subjects showed that perceived health status and locus of control were independently predictive of 2 or more of those health practices examined.

303. Stahl S. (1990). The Legacy of Longevity. Newbury Park, CA: Sage Publications.

Social gerontologists share state-of-the-art research on health and longevity. The implications of living longer and its impact on the quality of life of our older citizens are discussed. Topics explored include health promotion/disease prevention, governmental and community response to elder needs, and the effects of gender and ethnicity on health and life circumstances.

304. Stevenson J. S., Topp R. (1990). Effects of moderate and low intensity long-term exercise by older adults. Res Nurs & Health, 13(4):209-218.

Findings indicate that any level of exercise, according to client's physical abilities, prolongs independent functioning, and promotes positive perceptions of well-being in older adults.

305. Streib G. F. (1989). Retirement as seen by the health professional and the social scientist. In Clinical Aspects of Aging, 3rd Ed. W. Reichel (Ed.) Baltimore: Williams and Wilkins:495-503.

Responses to retirement and assisting clients to adjust

to retirement are the major emphases in this chapter. Research studies about adaptation to retirement show varying results in that people respond differently to retirement. Some adapt readily and find enjoyment in retirement activities apart from previous positions and type of work, while others no not adjust so easily, with resulting higher stress levels. Variables that affect adaptation ability relate to personality type, readiness to retire, and level of activities outside of work in which clients were engaged prior to retirement. Recommended for social workers, practitioners, researchers. families, and policy planners.

306. Tennant K. F. (1990). Laugh it off: The effect of humor on the well-being of the older adult. J Geront Nurs, 16(12):11-17.

Following a three-week humor program, older adults showed an increase in the post-test morale scores. The change in scores was sufficient to indicate support for the research hypothesis. The researcher cites several limitations of the study and recommends replication.

307. U.S. Congress, Office of Technology Assessment (1988). Mapping Our Genes: Genome Projects--How Big, How Fast? Baltimore: Johns Hopkins University Press.

Every health care professional needs to be concerned with the results being produced by the genome projects currently under way in this and other countries. Economic, social, and ethical aspects of these projects are discussed. Of greatest concern to health care professionals dealing with clients is the use of these research findings in drafting policies about an area that is far ahead technologically. Careful thought and consideration will be needed to develop appropriate policies on which to base future actions of health care providers. Recommended for geneticists, ethicists, and policy planners.

308. Weissert W. G., Cready C. M., Pawelak J. E. (1989). Home and community care: Three decades of findings. In Health Care of the Elderly. M. D. Petersen,

D. L. White (eds.). Newbury Park, CA: Sage Publications.

This chapter is a summary of the results of home and community care studies conducted since 1960. Studies included tested effects of providing home and community-based alternatives to existing long-term care services. Each study had at least 50 subjects, used an experimental design that included treatment and control groups, and used as the unit of analysis individuals who were providing care to elderly populations. Conclusions about costs and effects of home and community care of the elderly are discussed.

309. Williams B. C., Mackay S. A., Torner J. C. (1991). Home health care: comparison of patients and services among three types of agencies. Med Care, 29(6):583.

A substantial number of elderly Americans currently requires supportive services at home, and this number is expected to increase rapidly in the decades ahead. Medicare-certified home health agencies provide 50% to 70% of home care of all types, and a substantial part of all skilled home health services. Although Medicare regulations for these home health agencies are uniform, the agencies differ in organization and structure. Findings showed that hospital-based agencies substitute days of home health care for days of inpatient care, proprietary agencies operate to maximize revenue, and public agencies disproportionately serve poor and chronically ill patients.

7

Ethics

310. Annas G. J. (1989). The Rights of Patients: The Basic ACLU Guide to Patient Rights, 2nd Ed. Carbondale, IL: Southern Illinois University Press.

An excellent guide for health care professionals and for clients in terms of their rights as patients in any setting. Included in the discussion are topcis on informed consent, human experimentation, organ donation and transplantation, confidentiality, access to medical records, care of the dying, and other relevant concerns of both patients and care providers.

311. Baird R. M., Rosenbaum S. E. (eds.) (1989). Euthanasia: The Moral Issues. Buffalo, NY: Prometheus Books.

Controversies surrounding mercy killing are addressed in 19 well-written essays by physicians and ethicists. Included are discussions concerning assisted suicide, euthanasia as it is practiced in the Netherlands, sancity of life, infanticide, and the Karen Quinlan and Dax Cowart cases. Recommended for health professionals and others who provide care and counseling to clients and their families in situations where euthanasia may be a matter of conjecture.

312. Breckman R., Adelman R. (1988). Strategies for Helping Victims of Elder Mistreatment. Newbury Park, CA: Sage Publications - Sage Human Services Guides, Volume 53.

This helpful book provides suggestions for both assessment and interventions by health professionals. A comprehensive appendix includes a written protocol for identifying and assessing adult protective services referrals.

313. Brody B. A. (ed.) (1989). Suicide and Euthanasia: Historical and Contemporary Themes. Boston: Kluwer Academic Publishers.

Suicide and euthanasia are discussed by seven ethics philosophers in the context of historical philosophy. Reformation and Renaissance scholars, early Christians and Jews, and Greek philosophers are among those whose views are presented. Thought-provoking reading for all health care professionals, administrators, and policy planners.

314. Burt M. (1991). Face to face with bioethics: Health care providers thrust into cooperative effort. Aging Today:15, bimonthly newsletter of the American Society on Aging, Feb/Mar.

The experiences of a group of long-term care providers are discussed regarding their struggle to establish a systematic approach to bioethical dilemmas in their work with elderly clients. Although the setting is in nursing homes in California, the concepts and processes described are relevant to bioethical dilemmas encountered in any setting.

315. Collopy B., Dubler N., Zuckerman C. (1990). The ethics of home care: Autonomy and accommodation. Hastings Center Report, 20(2):S1-S16.

This report offers an exploration of home care and its distinctive ethical problems, particularly in the area of autonomy and allocation, specifically with respect to the frail elderly. Research was carried out by the Hastings Center and the Division of Legal and Ethical Issues in Health Care at Montefiore Medical Center. This research involved a comparative study of home care for the elderly and community-based care of the mentally ill. Ethical issues relevant to each, and to both, were described. Recommended for ethicists and researchers in the area of home care of the elderly.

316. Dejowski E. E. (1991). Protecting Judgment-Impaired Adults. Binghamton, NY: Haworth Press.

Valuable information is provided on guardianship and alternative methods for furnishing services to judgment-impaired adults, often the elderly. An array of topics is presented from several perspectives, including geographic insights about how these concepts of guardianship law and practice will be considered in the coming decades.

317. Faden R., Kass N. (1990). AIDS will pose moral dilemmas well into the 1990s. Kennedy Institute of Ethics Newsletter, 4(3), July. Washington, DC: Georgetown University.

Controversy in health care politics/policy regarding AIDS in our society is discussed in a thought-provoking way. The challenge for doctors and nurses in terms of their unconditional commitment and moral duty to their patients is addressed. The great strain being placed on an already overburdened health care system, the need for policies regarding health care insurance and employment rights of persons with AIDS (PWAs), and the concern to avoid discriminatory practices in the development of policies are addressed. Recommended for health professionals, policy planners, lawyers, and others interested in this major problem.

318. Fulmer T. T., O'Malley T. A. (1987). Inadequate Care of the Elderly: A Health Care Perspective on Abuse and Neglect. New York: Springer Publishers.

Abuse of older people is a common problem in our society. This book outlines methods of identifying the various types of abuse and neglect, and suggests interventions that can alleviate the situation. Legal and ethical issues are discussed, and ways are outlined by which legislation can assist in problem identification and reporting.

319. Graber G., Thomasma D. (1990). Euthanasia: Toward an Ethical Social Policy. New York: Continuum Press.

The authors develop a premise that today, there is little need for active euthanasia if more attention is paid to controlling pain and suffering, and to the patient's value system. If providers can give more specific responses to patients' requests to die, and if plans are made with the patient's family about the best way to bring about a kind and merciful death, the issue can be resolved well for all concerned. A problem arises only when the system does not work properly. Many perspectives are included for the purpose of presenting all sides to this controversial area, to allow reasoned and logical decisions to be made in a timely way.

320. Gunderson M., Mayo D., Rhame F. S. (1989). AIDS: Testing and Privacy. Salt Lake City: University of Utah Press.

Background information on AIDS medical history and aspects of privacy law are provided in the introduction. Specific issues with respect to testing are addressed and include AIDS education, insurer-employer, state-mandated, and voluntary anonymous testing, warning of patients and their partners, potential risks in health care delivery, and other relevant aspects of this complex problem.

321. Hackler C., Mosely R., Vawter D. E. (eds.) (1989). Advance Directives in Medicine. New York: Praeger Publishing Company.

An impressive array of essays cover various aspects of advance directives for clients. Included are the interpretation of proxy directives, financial endorsement of living wills, living will statutes, talking with clients about advance directives, health care for the elderly, and self-determination. Highly recommended for all health care professionals, administrators, and policy planners concerned with these issues.

322. The Hastings Center. (1988). Guidelines on the Termination of Life-Sustaining Treatment and the Care of the Dying. Bloomington, IL: Indiana University Press.

These guidelines have particular relevance in care of the elderly and in the support of their families and caregivers. As technology advances and the use of extraordinary means to prolong life becomes more usual, these guidelines will become even more important in the ethical decision making process that health care professionals and families must sometimes undertake. A must resource book for all practicing health care professionals in all settings. Caregivers and care providers in the home will find it particularly helpful.

323. Hogstel M. O., Gaul A. L. (1991). Safety or autonomy: An ethical issues for clinical gerontology nurses. J Geront Nurs, 17(3):6-11.

The family dilemma of deciding whether to force an elderly parent to move to a safer environment poses ethical questions of autonomy, benificence, nonmalfeasance, and justice for all concerned. Each situation must be considered on its own characteristics.

324. Loewy E. H. (1989). Textbook of Medical Ethics. New York: Plenum Medical Book Company.

A separate section of excellent case studies is included in this outstanding book. Ethical issues addressed include the patient/health care system, professional relationships, care of the terminally ill, organ donation, and the allocation of scarce resources to cover costs of health care. All of these questions are presented in a problem-solving way to guide discussion and help draw conclusions based on sound reasoning and experience. A history and theory of bioethics is introductory to the basic text.

325. Meisel A. (1989). The Right to Die. New York: John Wiley & Sons Publishers.

The right to die is defined by utilization of judicial

cases and statutes to explore the ethical and legal rights of individuals to die. A thorough explanation of the "right to die" issues are described. How decisions are generally made, the use of advance directives, and the role of ethics committees are discussed. Highly recommended for families and caregivers to the terminally ill or elderly.

326. Menzel P. T. (1990). Strong Medicine: The Ethical Rationing of Health Care. New York: Oxford University Press.

The effects of rationing of health care with equity are examined in this text. Included in the discussions are issues such as organ procurement and allocation, determining equity between the haves and the have-nots, measuring the quality of life, and the costs of utilizing extraordinary treatments to save lives and to prolong life. A thought-provoking book about major issues facing our entire society, particularly health care providers and policy decision makers.

327. Monagle J. F., Thomasma D. C. (eds.) (1988). Medical Ethics: A Guide For Health Professionals. Rockville, MD: Aspen Publishers, Inc.

This is a comprehensive volume on medical ethical issues that are addressed by experts in the field. An especially good chapter (32) on Quality Assurance, Risk Management, and Ethics is provided. The need to discuss all ethical issues in a systematic way by using basic ethical review criteria is emphasized in order to generate a patient management analysis that directs the needed corrective action. Excellent information on all aspects of ethics in relation to care of patients in all settings. Recommended for health care professionals, lawyers dealing with relevant cases, and interested others.

328. Pellegrino E. D., Veatch R. M., Langan J. P. (eds.) (1991). Ethics, Trust, and the Professions. Washington, DC: Georgetown University Press.

Essays on the philosophical and cultural aspects of

trust and ethics in the professions are presented in this volume. The professions particularly cited include medicine, law, and the ministry. The question regarding whom we can trust, and how far, is addressed. This collection is a result of an international conference on professional ethics held during Georgetown University's Bicentennial celebration in 1989. Three of the essays provide cross-cultural perspectives on the question of the fiduciary relationship by considering the perspectives of Japanese, Chinese, and European philosophers and ethicists.

329. Portenoy R. K. (ed.) (1991). Medical ethics: Physician-assisted suicide and euthanasia. J Pain & Symptom Management, 6(5):279-339.

This special issue comprises nine articles by experts on the subject of physician-assisted suicide and euthanasia as these relate to medical ethics. Topics include Liberty (privacy) and assisted suicide, Relationship between pain and symptom management to patient requests for physician-assisted suicide, Euthansasia: the way we do it, the way they do it (U.S., Germany, and The Netherlands), and The challenge for future debate on euthanasia. These topics and others, all from different perspectives, will be of interest to physicians, nurses, families, ethicists, and others.

330. Robb R. B. (1991). Growing Up, vol. 1. Binghamton, NY: Haworth Press.

The importance of the spiritual life in aging is highlighted in this volume. Health care professionals providing comprehensive care to a growing elderly population need to be aware of the importance of spirituality in an aging society. While the book is intended for congregations, pastors, and other kinds of spiritual advisors, it provides meangingful information for anyone who has the best interests of their elderly patients at heart.

331. Roybal E. R. (1991). Elder abuse: America's hidden crisis. Caring, 10(5):22-24.

For a variety of reasons elder abuse is less likely to be observed or reported than child abuse. Some of the reasons are fear of retribution by the caregiver, shame in having to report one's own family members, and the fact that many elderly are more often homebound and not out among other people. Also, people outside do not want to believe that such a dehumanizing problem exists. Making others aware of actions that are actual or potential continuing events is the responsibility of health care professionals and others who may suspect abuse or neglect.

332. Rozovsky F. A. (1990). A Consent to Treatment: A Practical Guide, 2nd Ed. Boston: Little, Brown and Company.

A rich appendix is included which provides copies of long and short consent forms, a consent checklist form, Jehovah's Witness cards and release forms, the Uniform Brain Death Act, and the Uniform Anatomical Gift Act. Consent for treatment in various situations is discussed in the twelve chapters. Major topics addressed include refusal of treatment, human experimentation, autopsy, organ donation, and involvement with various populations such as prisoners, children, mentally incompetent, and the elderly. Highly recommended for health care professionals, lawyers, social workers, and others who work with clients in these situations.

333. Silva M. C. (1990). Ethical Decision Making in Nursing Administration. Norwalk, CT: Appleton & Lange Publishing Company.

This book is the result of a five-year grant from the Division of Nursing, Bureau of Health Professions, Health Resources and Services Administration, to provide continuing education to nurse executives in ethical decision making knowledge and skills. Case studies presented by the participants are included and address a wide range of ethical dilemmas faced by nurses in diverse practice settings. Sections about care of elderly persons are valuable for health professionals and home care workers.

334. Steinmetz S. K. (1988). Duty Bound: Elder Abuse and Family Care. Newbury Park, CA: Sage Publications.

This book provides valuable insights into the world of the caregiver. Numerous references to interviews with caregivers illustrate their feelings, perceived burdens, and how they manage to cope with what often appear to be insurmountable obstacles. The content leads the reader to understand how abuse of the elderly can occur. Recommended for social workers, care providers, lawyers, and researchers.

335. Wertz D. C., Fletcher J. C. (eds.) (1989). Ethics and Human Genetics: A Cross-Cultural Perspective. New York: Springer-Verlag Publishing Company.

Ethical problems in medical genetics are discussed within the framework of results from a 19-nation survey. Chapters are contributed by medical ethicists and geneticists from each of the countries surveyed. Included in the discussion are topics regarding counseling, genetic screening, abortion, prenatal diagnosis, and the provision of other genetic services. This global perspective is excellent as a comparative resource book.

8

Care of the Terminally Ill

336. Blank J. J., Clark L., Longman A. J., Atwood J. R. (1989). Perceived home care needs of cancer patients and their caregivers. J Cancer Nurs, 12(2):78-84.

The purpose of this study was to identify perceived home care needs of outpatients receiving treatment for cancer, and needs of their caregivers. Stressors in their situation perceived by the patients included coping with physical restrictions that resulted in anger and depression. Caregivers' stressors centered mainly on the added burden and responsibilities of caring for cancer patients. Excellent resource for understanding interpersonal aspects of patients and caregivers.

337. Cohen C. B. (ed.) (1988). Casebook on the Termination of Life-Sustaining Treatment and the Care of the Dying. Bloomington, IL: Indiana University Press.

Ethical, medical, and legal dilemmas are discussed in this book, focused primarily on issues surrounding the decision to terminate treatment for the dying person. Twenty-six case studies provide the basis for discussion by experts in all fields. The content can be used to develop educational classes.

338. Dush D. M., Cassileth B. R., Turk D. C. (1987). Psychosocial Assessment in Terminal Care. Binghamton, NY: Haworth Press.

While the focus of this book is hospice care, the same principles of assessment and measurement of psychosocial aspects of terminal illness can be used with older persons being cared for in the home.

339. Harriet (1979). 16 mm film or 1/2" videocassette, 10 minutes, color. Available from Mass Media Ministries, 2116 N. Charles Street, Baltimore, MD 21218.

This documentary profile of a minister's wife, suddenly widowed, is one of a series of five films focusing on change, loss, and grief. Harriet recalls her feelings before and after her husband's death, which occurred at the same time that her adult children were leaving home. An especially effective teaching film that includes a teaching guide. Recommended for health care professionals, social workers, clergy, and those who counsel grieving persons.

340. Haskell G. W., Satter N. F. et al (1988). AIDS Home Care and Hospice Manual. San Francisco Visiting Nurses and Hospice.

This is a companion volume to Developing AIDS Residential Settings: A Manual, by the same authors. It is intended to train volunteers and direct-care providers in caring for AIDS patients in their homes. A companion video is also available for training purposes. Health care planners and providers will find this a useful resource.

341. Johnson I. S., Cockburn M., Pegler J. (1988). The Marie Curie/St. Luke's Relative Support Scheme: A home care service for relatives of the terminally ill. J Advanc Nurs, 13(5):565-70.

A hospice-based scheme for the support of relatives of dying patients is described. The majority of caregivers were female and almost a third were elderly. Most patients were suffering from malignancy. Caregivers reported a high level of satisfaction with the help they received from the program, but late referral was a common source of dissatisfaction. Emphasis was on volunteers' susceptibility to stress.

342. Montgomery Hospice Society, Bethesda, MD (1990). Hospice Services for Patients Without Caregivers. Washington, DC: Policy Information Center, ID# 2514.

Hospice clients without primary caregivers or family were provided services designed to compensate for their missing family in order to determine the feasibility of such a system of care. The report concludes that the concept is feasible so long as clients designate a reliable surrogate to make legal, medical, and financial decisions on their own behalf. Special problems in this situation are discussed in detail.

343. Parry J. K. (1989). Social Work: Theory and Practice With the Terminally Ill. Binghamton, NY: Haworth Press.

Case studies are used to assist health care professionals in their work with dying persons and their families. Impending death, financial worries, job concerns, pain, unfinished business, and spiritual needs are some of the topics identified as important during this time.

344. Rakel R. E., Storey P. (1990). Care of the dying patient. In Textbook of Family Practice, 4th Ed. R. E. Rakel (ed.). Philadelphia: W. B. Saunders Company, 181-197.

This concise chapter includes many of the issues and problems encountered in caring for terminally ill patients, with attitudes of care providers included at the beginning. Other topics are: communications, pain control management of symptoms, and measures such as subcutaneous infusions of fluids to prevent dehydration. Comprehensive, clinically based resource.

345. Rhymes J. A. (1991). Clinical management of the terminally ill. Geriatrics, 46(2):57-67.

More terminally ill patients are being cared for at

home. Although alleviating the disease condition is not possible, the patient's comfort and quality of life can be enhanced, and the degree of control they have over their own care can be maximized. Caregivers need to provide adequate communication regarding advance directives, and planning for death. Useful resource.

346. Stern M. (ed.) (1991). Psychotherapy and the Widowed Patient. Binghamton, NY: Haworth Press.

This book presents different approaches to bereavement and focuses specifically on the widowed client and on the helping professions. Methods and approaches described include psychoanalytic, humanist, existentialist, and cognitive. The variety of approaches to therapy provides valuable choices, and the counselor can use one or all.

9

Education of Caregivers

347. Assistance Services for the Elderly: Reference Book and Student Activity Book, (1988). ERIC no. ED 306386.

The reference book and student activity book describe the career cluster of assistance services for the elderly, including home health aides, and were developed by Texas Tech University at Lubbock. The reference book is designed for employees and includes a list of the most important and relevant competencies for caregivers to have. Unit tests and answer keys are provided. The books are correlated.

348. Brown P. (1986). Development of Home Health Aide Curriculum Project. Final Report. ERIC #ED 275808.

This report from Tacoma Community College, Washington, describes a curriculum for community college students that meets state requirements for nurse aide certification. This report includes outlines, objectives, and outcomes of the project to prepare home health aides.

349. A Guide for Planning Competency-Based Institutional and Home Management Services Education in Home Economics Education Programs. ERIC, no. ED 298306.

This guide from the South Carolina State Department of Education, Columbia, assists teachers in developing a competency-based vocational education program in occupational home economics emphasizing home health aides or homemaker services for the elderly. The plan comprises five units, and each includes performance objectives, guides, suggested learning experiences, and instructional resources.

350. Humphrey C. J. (1986). Home Care Nursing Handbook. Norwalk, CT: Appleton-Century-Crofts.

This handbook is a compact and practical guide written for home care nurses. The appendix contains valuable charts and tables that can be easily referenced to interpret symptoms and assist patients and families to plan appropriate care. The text includes discussion about the health care system as it relates to home care, and specific procedures for conditions commonly found in elderly persons being cared for at home.

351. Jung F. D. (1991). Teaching registered nurses how to supervise nursing assistants. J Nurs Admin, 21(4):31-36.

Nurse administrators are increasing their use of nursing assistants in all settings. This level of health care worker is called home health aides when the setting is the home. Many nurses who direct these assistants, however, have little knowledge or experience in personnel management. The author describes a program to improve nursing assistant supervision and discusses how the program has led to improved distribution of work load, and increased nursing assistants' productivity. Principles can be extrapolated to any setting.

352. Kadushin A. (1990). The Social Work Interview: A Guide for Human Service Professionals, 3rd ed. New York: Columbia University Press.

This new edition provides up-to-date information about methods of interviewing clients receiving services in any setting. New information is included on cross-ethnic interviewing, nonverbal aspects of interpersonal behavior, and on the use of a range of technical interviewing skills. Research is examined on ethnomethodology of face-to-face interactions. The use of computers is discussed in direct interviewing, and in processing information. Useful guide for developing interviewing techniques.

353. La-Mothe D. et al (1987). Homemaker/Home Health Aide. ERIC #ED-287034.

This document is a curriculum guide from the Arizona State Department of Education in Phoenix for vocational instruction for entry-level employment as homemaker/home health aides. It includes a competency and task list, an annotated bibliography, and an instructor's guide.

354. Martinson I. M., Widner A. (eds.) (1989). Home Health Care Nursing. Philadelphia: W. B. Saunders Company.

This textbook contains chapters on multiple aspects of home care, including discharge planning, reimbursement, symptom control and pain management, medication management, rehabilitation, ethical dilemmas, professional nursing issues, and specific disorders common in elderly persons. The book is a valuable reference for health care providers.

355. Nurse Assistant Instructor Guide, (1988). ERIC #ED-306462.

This document from the Connecticut State Department of Education in Hartford covers nine units and 72 lessons designed to prepare students for entry-level employment with a licensed home health care agency. It is a 135-hour course that prepares students to assist RNs or LPNs with direct patient care.

356. Robinson K. M. (1988). A social skills training program for adult caregivers. Advances in Nurs Sci, 10(2):59-72.

A model for family caregiving was developed that linked social support and caregiving burden. A component of the theoretical model suggests that caregivers with high social skills will be able to mobilize social support in their environments more effectively, resulting in a decrease of their perceived caregiving burden. Results revealed a significant decrease in both subjective and objective burden in the treatment group. Implications are disscussed regarding the importance of further research on how best to support caregivers.

10

Information

357. Administration on Aging (1991). Aging America - Trends and Projections. Washington, DC: Office of Management and Policy.

The 1991 edition of this publication will be available soon. This report is the first update to be issued since the 1987-88 edition, and is a joint report of the Administration on Aging, the American Association of Retired Persons, the U.S. Senate Special Committee on Aging, and the Federal Council on Aging. The paper is a compilation of the most current data on a wide variety of subjects and includes projections into the future for many topics. Some topics included are: 1) Size and Growth of the Older Population; 2) Economic Status; 3) Retirement Trends and Labor Force Participation; 4) Health Status and Health Services Utilization; 5) Long-Term Care; 6) Social Characteristics; 7) Elderly People Who Live Alone; 8) Federal Outlays Benefiting the Elderly; and 9) International Comparisons. A single copy at no charge may be obtained by contacting: Administration on Aging, Office of Management and Policy, Aging America: Trends and Projections, 330 Independence Avenue, SW, Washington, DC 20201, or calling 202/619-2614.

358. Audio-Visual Guide: Resources in Gerontology and Geriatrics. Los Angeles: Pacific Geriatric Education Center.

This publication is in its third edition and is now available for purchase. It is a comprehensive listing of interdisciplinary resource materials with new international and ethnicity components. Information is listed and provided for over 1000 gerontological and geriatric audiovisuals. To obtain information about the publication, write to Pacific Geriatric Education Center, 2250 Alcazar, CSC136, Los Angeles, CA 90033, or call 213/342-2064.

359. BESS - Benefits Eligibility Screening Service. A computer software program available from the United Seniors Health Coop, 1331 H Street, NW, Suite 500, Washington, DC 20005.

This software package provides information about entitlement programs for which older persons are likely eligible, with addresses and telephone numbers for each program.

360. Caregiver's Guide. Administration on Aging, U.S. Department of Health and Human Services, 330 Independence Avenue, SW, Washington, DC 20201. Also available from: Superintendent of Documents, Government Printing Office, Washington, DC, 20402.

This booklet provides helpful information to caregivers who are assuming the role for the first time and are seeking help in carrying out the many tasks and responsibilities that usually accompany this position.

361. Corbin D. E., Metal-Corbin J. (1991). Reach For It, 2nd ed. Cost - about $29.95. Available from Eddie Bowers Publishing Company, 2600 Jackson Street, Dubuque, IA 52001.

This handbook contains information on health, exercise, and dance for older adults. The second edition has new chapters on nutrition, sexuality, drugs, the aging body, and water exercises. Includes sample medical forms and fitness assessment. Valuable resource for older persons concerned with maintaining optimum health.

362. Crim S. (1988). Employers and Eldercare. Washington, DC: Bureau of National Affairs.

This booklet offers information about various ways that employers are responding to the needs of employees who are also responsible for the care of aging parents or spouse.

363. Family Caregivers of the Aging Program. Membership fee: about $25.00 per year. National Council on Aging (NCOA), Family Caregiver Program, 600 Maryland Avenue, SW, Washington, DC 20024.

364. A Handbook About Care in the Home, (1989). ERIC no. ED 312 566.

This handbook from the American Association of Retired Persons describes the concept of home care, available services, and the agencies that provide them. Glossary of home care terms included.

365. Killeffer E. H., Bennett R., Gruen G. (1985). Handbook of Innovative Programs for the Impaired Elderly. Binghamton, NY: Haworth Press.

A source of ideas about physical and occupational therapy programs for impaired elderly, discussing physical activity and rehabilitation and community linkage programs. Discusses incremental exercises for gradually increasing strength and movement.

366. Making Wise Decisions for Long-Term Care, (1989). ERIC no. ED 312 567.

This booklet from the American Association of Retired Persons in Washington, DC, describes community services that may be available to elderly persons receiving care in the home. It provides descriptions of the resources and programs.

367. National Institute on Aging. The Resource Directory for Older People. Gaithersburg, MD: NIA Information Center: Directory, P.O. Box 8057, Gaithersburg, MD

20898-8057. One copy free.

This directory lists national organizations that offer social services, consumer advice, health information, legal aid, and other assistance to older Americans and their families. Federal agencies, professional societies, private groups, and voluntary programs are included. Useful resource.

368. Geriatric Education Centers (1991). Selected Materials Produced by Geriatric Education Centers. Rockville, MD: Health Resources and Services Administration.

This paper is an updated version of previous announcements about educational materials available from the network of Geriatric Education Centers (GECs) that have been supported by Federal funds since 1983. The purpose of these centers is to provide education and training opportunities in geriatrics for health professions educators and practitioners. The centers maintain resource clearinghouses and develop and disseminate curriculum and teaching materials. This publication lists only a few examples of available materials, with names, addresses, and telephone numbers of the GECs. To receive a copy, contact the GEC Coordinator, Bureau of Health Professions, 5600 Fishers Lane, Room 8-103, Rockville, MD 20857, or call 301/443-6887.

369. Weiss J. C. (1988). The "Feeling Great!" Wellness Program for Older Adults. Binghamton, NY: Haworth Press.

Participants in this program learn to improve their physical, emotional, and psychological well-being through a structured, phased program that addresses individuals' needs holistically.

370. Yahnke R. (1988). The Great Circle of Life: A Guide to Films on Aging. Owings Mills, MD: National Health Publishing.

This unique reference book, directed primarily to health care educators, presents a categorized listing of films about aging. Film topics include cultural images, documentaries, symbolic statements, intergenerational relationships, relationships in old age, and reactions to loss. Some critics indicate that some of the listed films do not portray aging in a realistic way, so careful screening by users is necessary.

Author Index

Numbers are citation entry numbers, not page numbers.

Subject Index

Numbers are citation entry numbers, not page numbers.

About the Compilers

The compilers are Nurse Consultants with the Division of Nursing, Bureau of Health Professions, Health Resources and Services Administration of the U.S. Public Health Service.

ADA ROMAINE-DAVIS held academic positions for 15 years before joining the federal government, and was associate dean of the graduate program, Georgetown University School of Nursing. An adult nurse practitioner, she has extensive practical and scholarly experience in home health care.

AYELIFFE A. LENIHAN has broad experience in the field of gerontology in practice, teaching, research, and publications. She held academic positions at George Mason University, developed the Assessment Tool to Identify Self-Care Behaviors in Community-Based Elderly, and is a consultant to universities and organizations regarding the elderly.

MOIRA D. SHANNON was a Health Scientist Administrator at the National Center for Nursing Research. She has held academic appointments at The Catholic University of America and George Mason University. She has conducted research and published in gerontology and home care.